Ultrasonography Diagnosis
of Peripheral Nerves

Dingzhang Chen • Minjuan Zheng

Editors

Ultrasonography Diagnosis of Peripheral Nerves

Cases and Illustrations

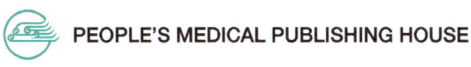 PEOPLE'S MEDICAL PUBLISHING HOUSE

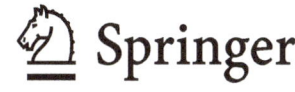 Springer

Editors
Dingzhang Chen
Department of Ultrasound
Xijing Hospital
Fourth Military Medical University
Xi'an
Shaanxi
China

Minjuan Zheng
Department of Ultrasound
Xijing Hospital
Fourth Military Medical University
Xi'an
Shaanxi
China

ISBN 978-981-15-2703-6   ISBN 978-981-15-2704-3   (eBook)
https://doi.org/10.1007/978-981-15-2704-3

This Springer imprint is published by the registered company Springer Nature Singapore Pte Ltd.
The registered company address is: 152 Beach Road, #21-01/04 Gateway East, Singapore 189721, Singapore

Foreword

Musculoskeletal ultrasound has become a valuable imaging method for its extensive clinical applications in orthopedics, sports medicine, rehabilitation therapy, pain management, anesthesia, and so on. High-resolution ultrasound imaging can be used to make accurate diagnoses of peripheral nerve diseases with its real-time approach. However, the anatomy of peripheral nerves is complex, with extensive distribution in the human body, running between muscles and blood vessels. This complexity requires the examiner to have rich anatomical and clinical knowledge. The correct diagnosis of peripheral nerve abnormalities can only be made by mastering the standard operating techniques and being familiar with typical sonographic characteristics of various lesions. Thus, a dedicated ultrasound textbook that covers the anatomy, physiology, and pathology of peripheral nerves in clinical examples, along with audio-video demonstration, will surely be favored and welcomed.

Professor Dingzhang Chen at Xijing Hospital of Air Force Medical University (formerly known as the Fourth Military Medical University) is a well-known musculoskeletal ultrasound expert in China, especially for peripheral nerve diseases. In 1996, Dr. Chen studied at Thomas Jefferson University Hospital and worked with me for a year. During his decades of dedication to ultrasound, Dr. Chen led his team to obtain tremendous basic and clinical achievements in ultrasound of the peripheral nervous system. Dr. Chen and his colleagues made great efforts to present this book in an audio-video format and illustrate a variety of common and typical cases involving peripheral nerves to the readers, which will certainly serve as extraordinary learning experiences. No doubt, the *Ultrasonography Diagnosis of Peripheral Nerves: Cases and Illustrations* will prove to be a useful tool of great benefit to learners.

Ji-Bin Liu
Jefferson Ultrasound and Radiology Education Institute
Thomas Jefferson University Hospital
Philadelphia, PA, USA

Preface

With the increased development of technologies, ultrasonic examination has become one of the most useful diagnostic modalities for the musculoskeletal system and is often used in parallel with X-ray, computed tomography (CT), and magnetic resonance imaging (MRI). It has been widely applied in the fields of orthopedics, hand surgery, pain management, immunology, physiotherapy, rehabilitation medicine, and neurology. In particular, high-resolution ultrasonography can provide high-quality imaging for most of the human peripheral nervous system and can even compete with MRI imaging in some cases. High-resolution ultrasonography has been considered a reliable examination method for clinical peripheral neurological diseases, but there are only a few books that focus on neurological ultrasonography. Therefore, I considered writing a simple, instructive professional book on neurological ultrasound based on my decades of experience and case studies.

I have engaged in the specialty of ultrasound for over 30 years. In 1996, I had the privilege of learning from Professor Barry Goldberg and Professor Liu Jibin, the international authorities on ultrasound at Thomas Jefferson University in Philadelphia. This was also the first time I had a preliminary understanding of the clinical application of musculoskeletal superficial ultrasound. When I returned to China in March 1998, I was invited to join the consultation on a patient who may have suffered from median nerve damage, during which a clinical hand surgeon asked me whether ultrasound could be used for examining nerves. Therefore, I made my first attempt to use ultrasound to visualize nerves and found the position of the neurological fracture, which led to the diagnosis; the surgery outcome later validated the same finding as the ultrasound. Since then, I began to work on the science of neurological ultrasound. With years of collaboration with my colleagues in the neurology and hand surgery departments, I have finally achieved today's accomplishments.

This book on case diagrams includes many anatomy diagrams from fresh corpses and operating rooms, and helps readers deeply understand the path through which nerves run. We collected a variety of ultrasound imaging data and surgical results covering different content, including the most common diseases and typical cases. This book, which contains ultrasound images and dynamic surgical videos with audio explanations, is easily understood; thus, this book is especially suited for doctors who are specialists in medical imaging, orthopedics, neurology, anesthesiology, pain management, and physiotherapy for rehabilitation.

Lastly, I would like to take this opportunity to thank my wife, Ms. Wang Danyun, for her support and contributions to our family. Without her help, I would not have had the spare time to complete this book alongside my busy schedule of clinical work. Additionally, I would like to express my gratitude to my team for their efforts in the preparation of this book.

Xi'an, China   Dingzhang Chen
May, 2019

The original version of the chapter has been revised. A correction to this chapter is available at https://doi.org/10.1007/978-981-15-2704-3_6

Acknowledgements

Mr. Qi Zhang and Mr. Chen Fan
Hitachi Medical (Guangzhou) Co., Ltd

Contents

Jing Wang, Dingzhang Chen, and Minjuan Zheng

1.1 Overview of the Anatomy of Peripheral Nerves

The peripheral nervous system refers to the neural structures and tissues throughout the body except the brain and spinal cord. The central nerves include 31 pairs of spinal nerves connected to the spinal cord and 12 pairs of cranial nerves connected to the brain. Peripheral nerves include somatic nerves at the body surface, bones, joints and skeletal muscles, and visceral nerves in the viscera, cardiovascular system, smooth muscles and glands.

As the basic unit of the peripheral nerve, nerve fibres consist of the long protuberance of a neuron and surrounding neurogliocytes. Aggregated nerve fibres each surrounded by endoneurium form a nerve fibre bundle in the perineurium, and different numbers of nerve fibre bundles surrounded by the epineurium form nerve trunks (Fig. 1.1) with branches spreading throughout the body. Nerve fibres in nerve trunks run through and between different fibre bundles, which causes

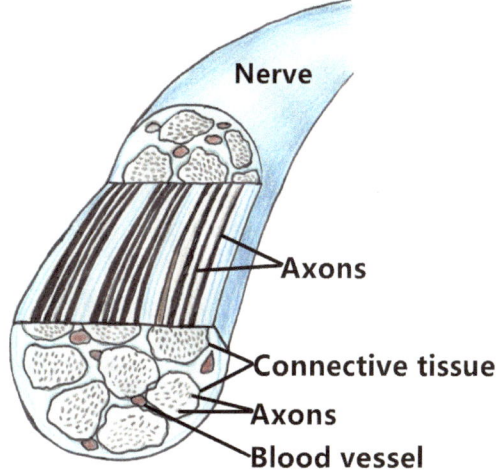

Fig. 1.1 Diagram of nerve patterns

variance in the size, number and position of fibre bundles. Except for nerve fibres, peripheral nerve trunks also include many interstitial tissues consisting of collagen fibres, elastic fibres, adipose tissues, blood vessels and lymphatic vessels. These interstitial tissues are primarily distributed among fibre bundles with a small amount in nerve bundles. The large number of interstitial tissues in nerve trunks leads to variance in the positions of fibre bundles in the trunks. Blood vessels supplying the nerve travel in the epineurium and branch into the perineurium and the endoneurium, where they form a capillary network.

Nerves share common characteristics in routing and distribution: larger nerve trunks run alongside blood vessels in the fascial sheath of

Supplementary Information The online version contains supplementary material available at https://doi.org/10.1007/978-981-15-2704-3_1.

J. Wang (✉) · D. Chen · M. Zheng
Department of Ultrasound, Xijing Hospital,
Fourth Military Medical University,
Xi'an, Shaanxi, China

the same connective tissue, where they form vascular nerve bundles, which are usually in the flexural sides of joints. Some nerves run without the accompaniment of blood vessels due to gradual degeneration during embryonic development [1].

1.2 Structures of the Main Peripheral Nerves in the Cervical Region and Limbs (Video 1.1)

ER 1.1 Systemic neuroanatomy

1.2.1 Brachial Plexus

The brachial plexus consists of the most fibres of the C5–8 and T1 anterior branches, which run into the axilla through the scalene muscle space and the posterosuperior part of the subclavian artery. The C5 and 6 anterior branches form the superior trunk, the C7 anterior branch continues in the middle trunk, and fibres at the C8 and T1 anterior branches form the inferior trunk. Each section of the trunk contains two nerves each in the anterior and posterior parts, which run into the axilla from the posteroinferior part of the middle section of the clavicle, which forms the medial, lateral and posterior cords (Figs. 1.2 and 1.3). The anaesthesia block position for a supraclavicular brachial plexus nerve block is the upper portion of the clavicle midpoint. The dorsal scapular nerve, subclavian nerve and long thoracic nerve branch at the superior brachial plexus clavicular portion. The brachial plexus and subclavian artery are surrounded by the fascial sheath formed by the prevertebral fascia and continues at the axillary sheath [2, 3] (Videos 1.2, 1.3, 1.4, 1.5, 1.6, and 1.7).

ER 1.2, ER 1.3, ER 1.4, ER 1.5, ER 1.6 and ER 1.7 Anatomy map of the brachial plexus and illustration

The surface projection of the brachial plexus is at the top 1/4 equally divided part of the straight-line section from the clavicle midpoint to the chelidon when the upper limbs are extended outward by 90°.

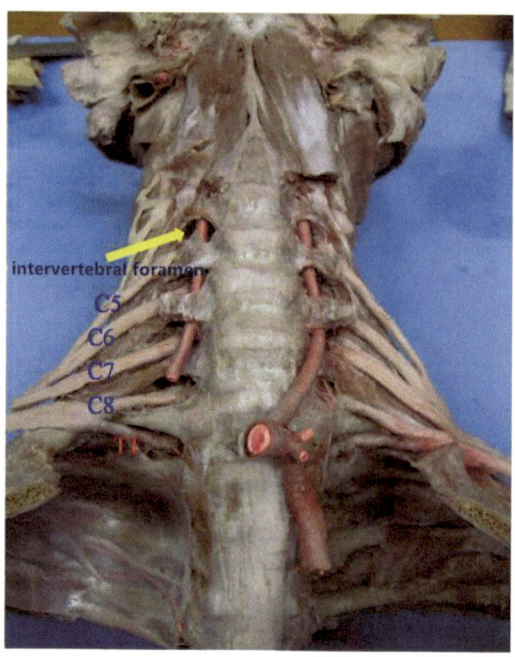

Fig. 1.2 Anatomy of the brachial plexus. Note: C5, C6, C7, C8 and T1 form the brachial plexus. The arrow points the intervertebral foramen, which contains a blood vessel (vertebral artery)

1.2.2 Median Nerve

(C6–T1) The medial branch of the medial cord and the lateral branch of the lateral cord from the brachial plexus converge at the anterior part of the axillary artery, as the median nerve trunk runs downward from the lateral side of the brachial artery to the end point of the coracobrachialis muscle. This covers the superficial surface or the deep surface of the brachial artery and turns to the inner side of the artery, going downward to the chelidon along with the blood vessel. The cord and blood vessel extend downward through the pronator teres muscle and the flexor superficialis tendon arch; they then travel downward at the median forearm and reach the wrist along the part between the flexor digitorum superficialis muscle and the flexor digitorum profundus muscle. The cord then travels through the carpal canal between the flexor carpi radialis muscle tendon and the palmaris longus tendon, where it branches on the deep surface of the palmar fascia and extends through the palm (Figs. 1.4, 1.5 and 1.6).

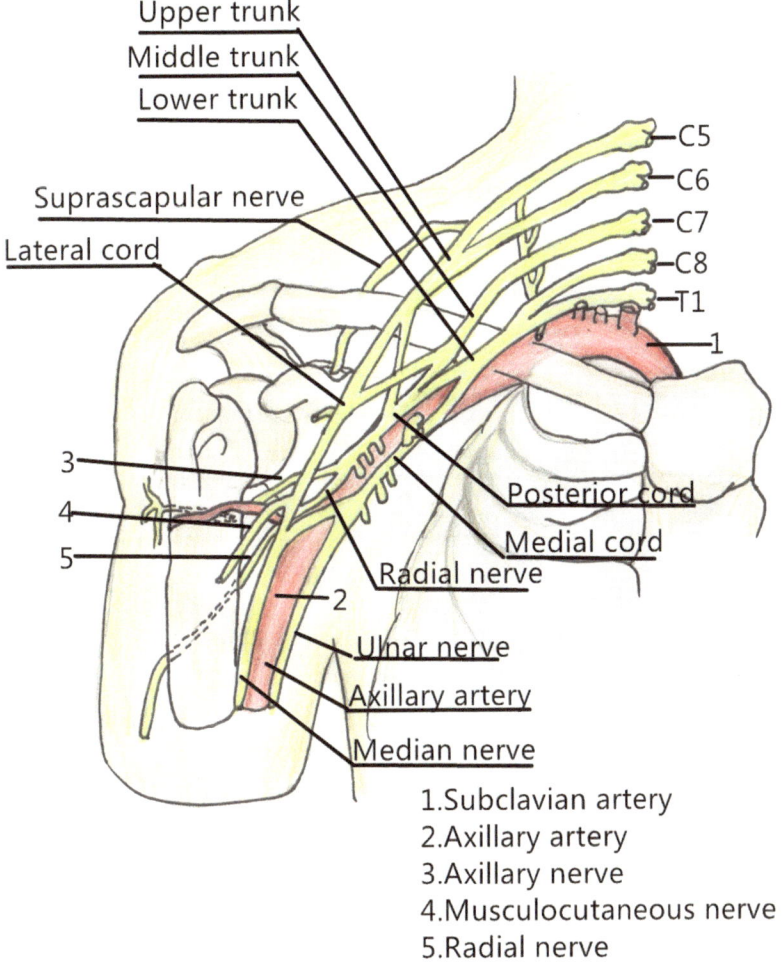

Upper trunk
Middle trunk
Lower trunk

C5
C6
C7
C8
T1
1

Suprascapular nerve

Lateral cord

3
4
5

Posterior cord
Medial cord
Radial nerve

2

Ulnar nerve

Axillary artery

Median nerve

1. Subclavian artery
2. Axillary artery
3. Axillary nerve
4. Musculocutaneous nerve
5. Radial nerve

Fig. 1.3 Anatomic diagram of the brachial plexus

Fig. 1.4 Anatomy of the upper arm nerves. Note: The white arrow indicates the ulnar nerve, the blue arrow indicates the median nerve and the black arrow indicates the musculocutaneous nerve

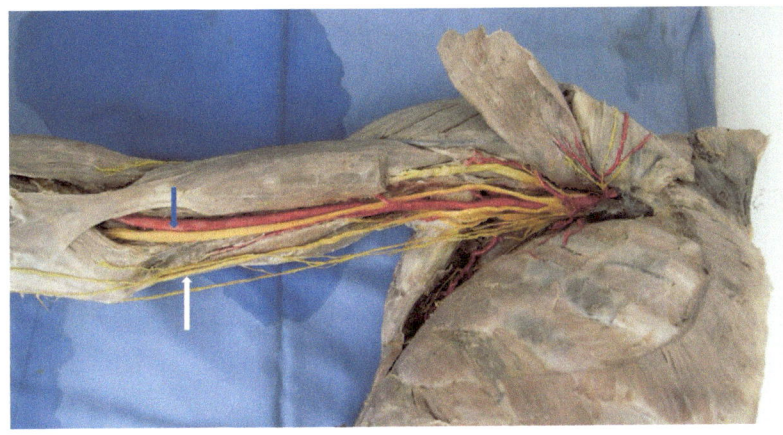

Fig. 1.5 Anatomy of the forearm nerves. Note: The white arrow indicates the ulnar nerve, the blue arrow indicates the median nerve and the black arrow indicates the radial nerve

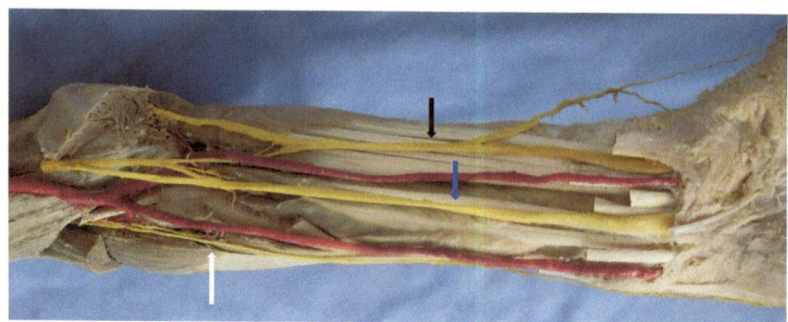

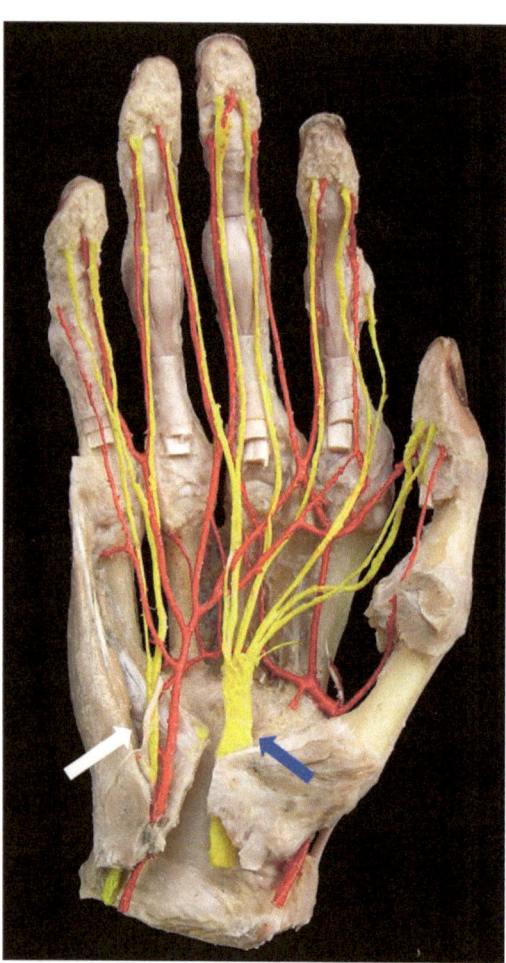

Fig. 1.6 Anatomy of the palmar nerves. Note: The white arrow indicates the superficial branch of the ulnar nerve and the blue arrow indicates the median nerve

The surface projection line for the upper arm median nerve is derived from the brachial artery pulse at the upper part of the medial bicipital sulcus to the nearly inner side of the midpoint between the medial and external epicondyles of the humerus. The projection line for the forearm median nerve can be obtained by extending the above projection line to the midpoint between the flexor carpi radialis muscle tendon and the palmaris longus tendon.

1.2.3 Ulnar Nerve

(C8–T1) Starts from the fasciculus medialis plexus brachialis, exits out of the armpit through the axillary artery and vein and runs down to the middle of the arm from the medial bicipital sulcus and the medial side of the brachial artery. It then travels to the medial side of the posterior brachial region through the medial intermuscular septum, down to the sulcus of the ulnar nerve at the rear of the medial epicondyle of the humerus. The nerve then runs through the starting point of the flexor carpi ulnaris to the anteromedial superficial zone from back to front and is accompanied by the ulnar artery down to the upper side of the radiocarpal joint between the flexor carpi ulnaris and the flexor digitorum profundus before coming out of the dorsal branch. Its stem is located at the radialis pisiform bone, and the superficial surface of the flexor retinaculum, which is divided into the superficial branch and the deep branch, moves into the palm through the deep surface of the palmar fascia and the superficial surface of the transverse carpal ligament.

Surface projection: the projection line of the ulnar nerve in the upper arm begins from the pulse point of the brachial artery at the inferior margin of the pectoralis major, with its medial area down to the line between the medial malleolus of the humerus and olecranon. The projection line of the ulnar nerve in the forearm extends this line at the ulnar side of the forearm to the outside of the pisiform bone. The ulnar nerve is located at the shallowest position of the sulcus of the ulnar nerve at the rear of the medial epicondyle of the humerus, and thus it is easily found.

1.2.4 Radial Nerve

(C5–T1) Located behind the axillary artery, exits the posterior cord of the brachial plexus and travels down and outward together with the deep brachial artery between the lateral head and the medial head of the triceps brachii. These nerves then move down from the outside behind the middle of the humerus along the radial groove, then through the lateral intermuscular septum on the slightly upper side of the external epicondyle of the humerus to between the brachialis and brachioradialis. The nerves travel further down between the brachioradialis and the extensor carpi radialis longus. Radial nerves spread out with many branches from the arms, among which muscular branches are mainly distributed at the triceps brachii, anconeus, brachioradialis and the extensor carpi radialis longus. Joint branches are primarily at the elbow joints, and there are three skin branches: cutaneous nerves behind the arms are mainly distributed within the skin at the rear of the arms after coming out of the armpits; cutaneous nerves in the lower parts of the lateral

sides of the arms are mainly distributed within the lower lateral skin of the arms after coming out dead centre from the deltoid muscle; cutaneous nerves behind the forearm move down to the rear of the forearm until they reach the wrists after coming out of the lateral side of the middle of the arm and are distributed within the skin behind the forearms.

Surface projection: the line that slants down from the outside at the junction of the lateral end of the inferior margin of the axillary fossa posterior and the arm until it connects with the external epicondyle of the humerus is the projection line of the radial nerve on the posterior surface of the upper arm.

1.2.5 Sciatic Nerve, Tibial Nerve and Common Peroneal Nerve

1. *The sciatic nerve* (L4, L5 and S1–S3), the largest and longest nerve in the human body, exits the pelvic cavity to the deep surface of the gluteus maximus from the infrapiriform foramen, down between the ischial tuberosity and the greater trochanter to the posterior region of the thigh. This nerve then travels further down from the deep surface of the long head of the biceps femoris muscle, and finally above the popliteal space where it branches into the tibial nerve and the common peroneal nerve (Figs. 1.7, 1.8 and 1.9). The sciatic sends out muscular branches to control the biceps femoris, semitendinosus and semimembranosus muscles, while other branches go to the hip joint.

   Surface projection: the upper 2/3 section from the centre between the ischial tuberosity and the greater trochanter down to the centre between the medial and lateral condyles of the thigh bone is the projection line of the sciatic nerve at the posterior region of the thigh. When sciatica occurs, patients will experience apparent tenderness in this section.

Fig. 1.7 Anatomy of the lower limb nerves (sciatic nerve, tibial nerve and common peroneal nerve). Note: white arrow indicates the tibial nerve, the blue arrow indicates the common peroneal nerve and the black arrow indicates the sciatic nerve

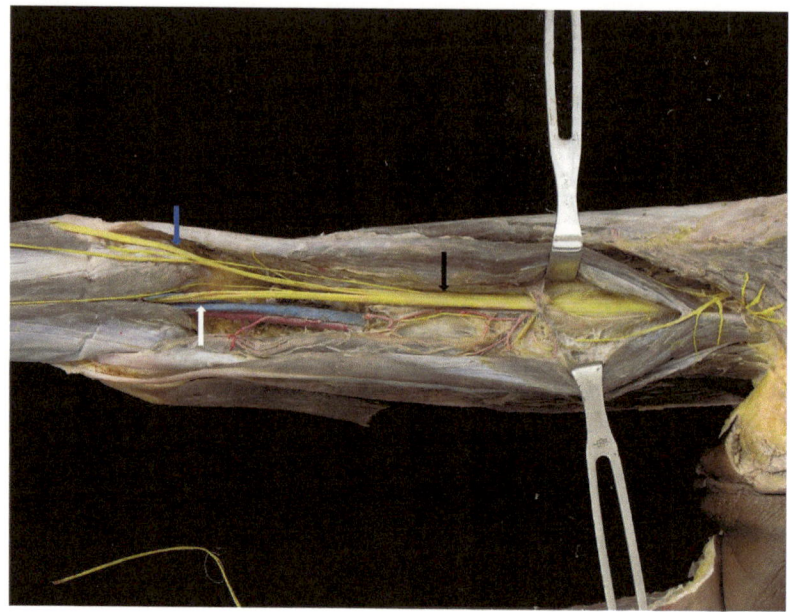

2. *The tibial nerve* (L4, L5 and S1–S3), the extension of the sciatic nerve stem, travels down into the popliteal space, further down to the rear of the crus and the deep surface of the soleus along with the popliteal vessels located on the deep surface. This nerve then runs to the rear of the medial malleolus together with the posterior tibial vessels, and finally into the bottom of the foot after it divides into the medial plantar nerves and the lateral plantar nerves in the tarsal tunnel with the deep surface supported by the flexor.

Surface projection: the line from the centre between the medial and lateral condyles of the thigh bone down to the downward straight line at the rear of the medial malleolus is the surface projection line of the tibial nerve.

3. *The common peroneal nerve* (L4, L5, S1 and S2), which divides into the superficial peroneal nerve and the deep peroneal nerve, exits the sciatic nerve near the popliteal space and travels down from the outside along the medial side of the muscle tendon of the biceps femoris to the lateral side of the upper crus. This

nerve then runs forward to the rear of the peroneus longus around the collum fibulae. The common peroneal nerve is vulnerable because of its shallow position at the collum fibulae.

Surface projection: the line from the upper corner of the popliteal space to the medial border of the biceps femoris and to the rear of the low fibular head is the projection line of the common peroneal nerve.

1.2.6 Femoral Nerve and Saphenous Nerve

The femoral nerve, the largest nerve from the lumbar plexus, exits the lateral border of the psoas major muscle and travels down between the psoas major muscle and the iliacus to the inguinal region. The nerve then runs through the slightly lateral side of the centre of the inguinal ligament and finally enters the area of the femoral triangle of the thigh from the lateral side of the femoral artery. The femoral nerve is divided into multiple branches from the area of the femoral

Fig. 1.8 Anatomy of
the lower limb nerves
(piriformis and sciatic
nerve). Note: white
arrow indicates the
sciatic nerve and the
blue arrow indicates the
piriformis

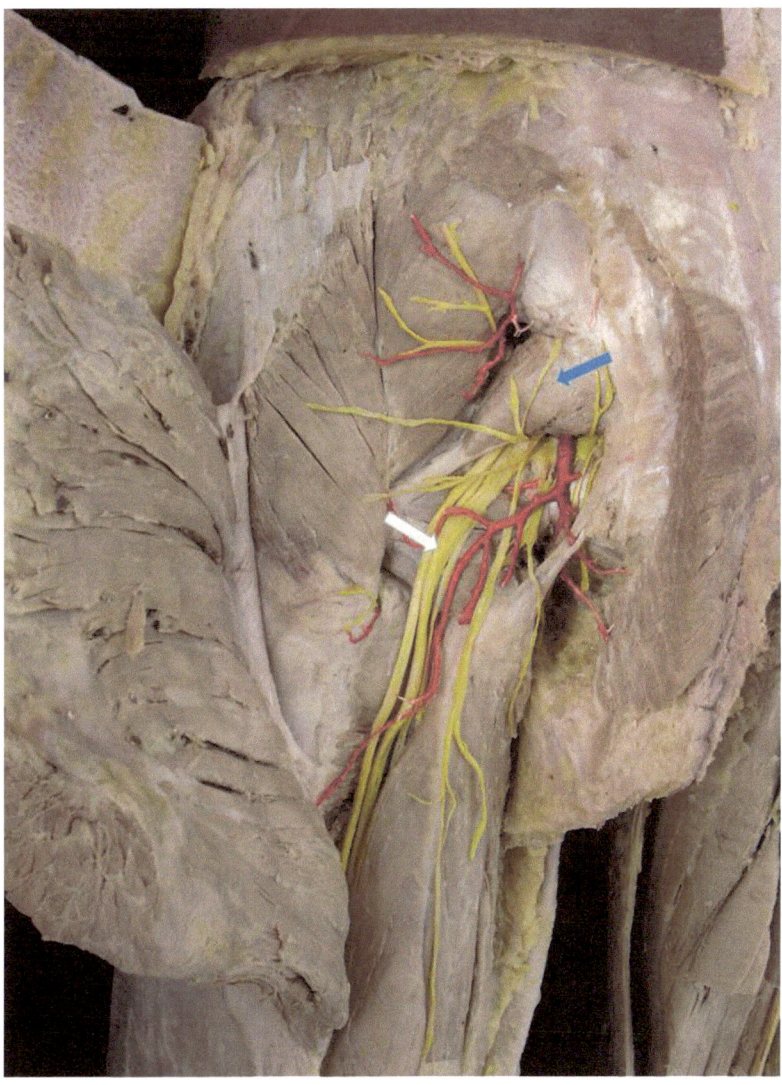

triangle, and among these, the muscular branches
are mainly distributed in the iliacus, pectineus,
quadriceps femoris and sartorius; skin branches
include the intermediate femoral cutaneous
nerves and the lateral femoral cutaneous nerves,
the routes of which are shorter throughout the
body and are distributed in the skin in the front
portions of the thighs and knees.

The saphenous nerve, the longest nerve in the
skin branch of the femoral nerve, travels downward until it exits the adductor canal after it
enters the adductor canal together with the femoral artery; this nerve then continues downward
at the medial side of the knees until it reaches
the subcutaneous tissues from the rear of the
lower sartorius muscle (Fig. 1.10). Then, it
travels, together with the great saphenous vein,
along the internal side of the crus down to the
medial border of the foot; it sends out branches
distributed in the skin under the kneecap, the

Fig. 1.9 Sciatic nerve and piriformis in a fresh corpse. Note: yellow arrow indicates the piriformis and the red arrow indicates the sciatic nerve

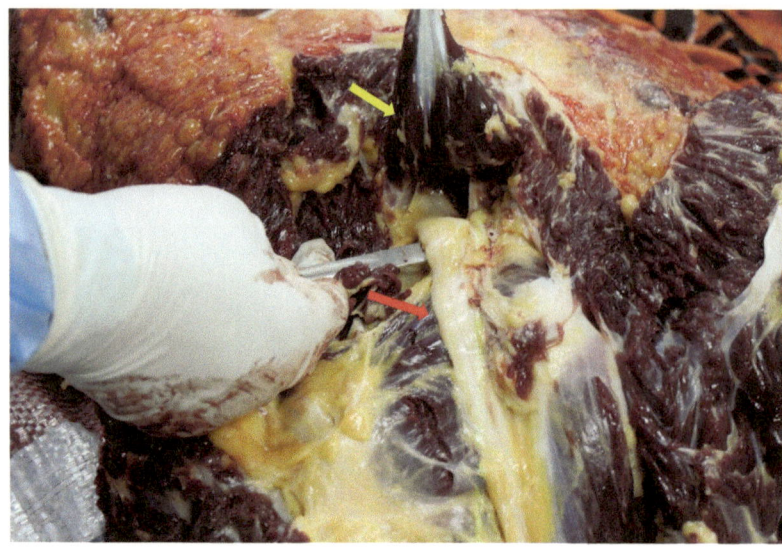

Fig. 1.10 Anatomy of the lower limb nerve (saphenous nerve). Note: blue arrow indicates the saphenous nerve

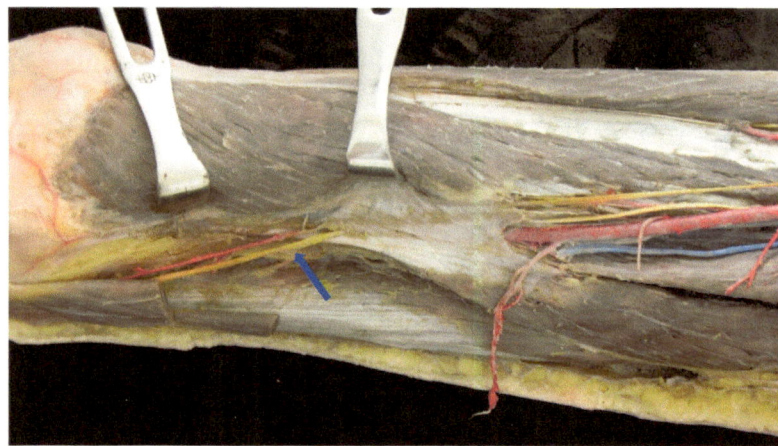

inner side of the crus and on the medial border of the foot [4, 5].

Surface projection: the 5-cm line that runs vertically from 1 cm (where the femoral nerve branches out from the inguinal ligament) outside the position of the femoral artery that passes behind the centre of the inguinal ligament and that can be felt is the surface projection line of the femoral nerve. The line from the inside of the knee to above the inside of the ankle along the medial border of the tibia is equivalent to the projection line of the saphenous nerve.

References

1. Wang J, Liu J. Musculoskeletal ultrasound. Beijing: Scientific and Technical Documentation Press; 2007.
2. Hong LY, Wang AP, Hong L, et al. Microanatomy of the brachial plexus roots and its clinical significance. Surg Radiol Anat. 2017;39(6):601–10.
3. Cui L. Atlas of peripheral nerve ultrasound. Beijing: Peking University Medical Press; 2004.
4. Wang Y. Fundamentals of musculoskeletal ultrasound. Beijing: Science Press; 2003.
5. Guo R. Musculoskeletal ultrasound. Beijing: People's Medical Publishing House; 2008.

Scanning Methods for Peripheral Nerves and Normal Ultrasonograms

2

Minjuan Zheng, Jing Wang, Dingzhang Chen, and Wenqing Gong

2.1 Scanning Methods

2.1.1 Preparation Before Examination

According to the different body parts to be scanned, the corresponding position in which patients feel comfortable and facilitates scanning is chosen without special preparation. A 10 MHz high-frequency linear probe is generally used for scanning, while a higher frequency probe is selected for superficial cutaneous nerves.

2.1.2 Examination Methods

Surface projection scanning along the route that the nerves run: horizontal and vertical scanning is performed on the short-axis cross section of the nerves to assess the neural structure; the probe

should then be rotated 90° to trace the long axis of the nerve for longitudinal scanning while paying heed to the identification of blood vessels, muscle tendons and ligaments.

2.1.3 Notes and Tips

What should be primarily observed during the examination of peripheral nerves includes the neural continuity, the changes in the neuromechanism and echoes, the relationships of the nerves to their adjacent masses and the dislocation of neural positions during joint movement [1–4].

Patients' medical histories should be known prior to neural ultrasonography to understand whether they have nerve stimulation symptoms in the corresponding innervation zones and to know about their activities or occupations as they relate to nerve entrapment. When it is doubted as to whether a nerve has a lesion, Tinel's test should be performed to judge neural irritation (Tinel's sign refers to a sort of electric shock-like numbness and pain or formication in its supportive dermatome when the position with the neural injury or lesion or its distal side is rapped, which represents the level of nerve regeneration or the position of the neural lesion).

Electromyography is an objective indicator that describes the potential of nerve-muscle conduction movement and is also a significant reference for ultrasonic examination [5].

Supplementary Information The online version contains supplementary material available at https://doi.org/10.1007/978-981-15-2704-3_2.

M. Zheng (✉) · J. Wang · D. Chen · W. Gong
Department of Ultrasound, Xijing Hospital,
Fourth Military Medical University,
Xi'an, Shaanxi, China

2.1.4   Adjustment of the Instrument

The medium- and high-quality colour Doppler ultrasound instrument that is generally used has relatively higher resolution and certain penetrability for superficial organs. The selected linear array probe has a frequency of 7–10 MHz, and if necessary, the 3.5 MHz sector-scanning probe can assist in examining deep tissues (for example, if the sciatic nerve needs to be examined in cases of thick thigh muscles).

2.2   Normal Ultrasonogram

A typical short-axis section for peripheral nerves is an oval structure with a mesh structure inside, where the hypoechoic area represents nerve bundles and the hyperechoic area is the spacing between nerve bundles. During long-axis section scanning, nerve bundles present as stripe-like hypoechoic structures, and they have a regular array with linear hyperechoic interstitial tissue. The epineurium presents as a linear hyperechoic structure. The ultrasonic characteristics of nerves, which are similar in nerves from different areas of the body but are not exactly the same, are affected by the probe frequency, the thickness of nerves and the incident angles of acoustic beams.

2.2.1   Brachial Plexus

The brachial plexus consists of the C5–C8 and T1 neural anterior branches, with C5 and C6 forming the superior trunk; C7 stretches to the middle trunk, and C8 and T1 constitute the inferior trunk on the surface of the scalenus minimus muscle. Each trunk has two nerves that are, on average, 1 cm in length in the anterior and posterior areas. The nerves in the anterior part of the superior and middle trunks form the lateral cord, the nerve in the anterior part of the inferior trunk directly stretches to the medial cord, and the nerves in the posterior parts of the three trunks constitute the posterior cord. Then, each bundle branches into the median nerve, radial nerve, ulnar nerve and axillary nerve in the upper limbs, which run along the subclavian artery and other artery branches.

Methods for scanning the brachial plexus: ultrasonic examination of the brachial plexus includes examinations of the nerve root, interscalene region, supraclavicular region, infraclavicular region and axillary region.

1. Nerve root: the root of the brachial plexus includes the C5, C6, C7, C8 and T1 nerves, but the root of the T1 nerve is deep, and thus it is not included in routine ultrasonic examinations. A short-axis ultrasonogram of the brachial plexus can be shown between the anterior scalene muscle and the middle scalene muscle, while a long-axis ultrasonogram can be shown by rotating the probe 90° (Figs. 2.1, 2.2 and 2.3). Each nerve root can be pinpointed as per the position where the vertebral artery runs into the cervical transverse foramen, and the shape of the cervical transverse process can also help determine the position of the brachial plexus nerve root. That is, the transverse processes of cervical vertebra C5 and C6 have an anterior tubercle and a posterior tubercle, which are shown as two nodular hyperechoic structures in the anterior and posterior areas on the ultrasonogram, with an acoustic shadow behind. The nerve root runs outward down from the groove between the anterior and posterior tubercles, and the cervical vertebra C7 only has a posterior tubercle (Fig. 2.4). According to such a feature, the 7th cervical vertebra and its corresponding C7 nerve root can be determined, while the other nerve roots can be successively confirmed horizontally to vertically (Figs. 2.5, 2.6 and 2.7). During examination of the cross section of the nerve, the probe can be transversely placed on one side of the neck to show the cervical nerve root structure between the anterior and posterior tubercles [6]; the examination is then performed on the vertical section (Videos 2.1, 2.2 and 2.3).

2. Interscalene region: the examinee is in the supine position, with the head towards one side. The probe is transversely placed on the lateral side of the neck, approximately 2 cm above the midclavicular line. The superior, middle and inferior trunks of the brachial plexus can be seen between the anterior and middle scalene muscles (see Fig. 2.8) and

Fig. 2.1 Short-axis ultrasonogram of the nerve root of the brachial plexus. Note: (**a**) shows C5, C6, C7 and C8 of the brachial plexus, *AS* anterior scalene muscle, *MS* middle scalene muscle; (**b**) is a scan of the brachial plexus nerve root

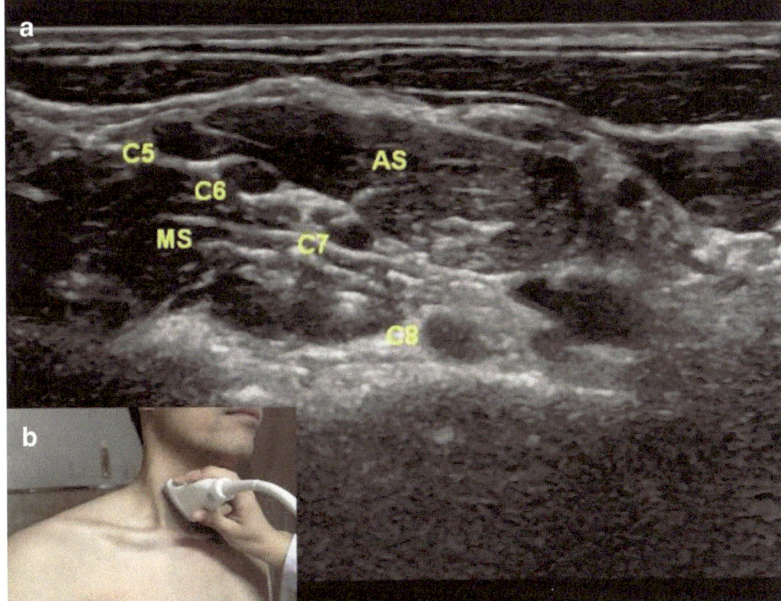

Fig. 2.2 Long-axis ultrasonogram of the brachial plexus nerve root. Note: *VA* vertebral artery; C5, C6 and C7 refer to the long axis of the brachial plexus

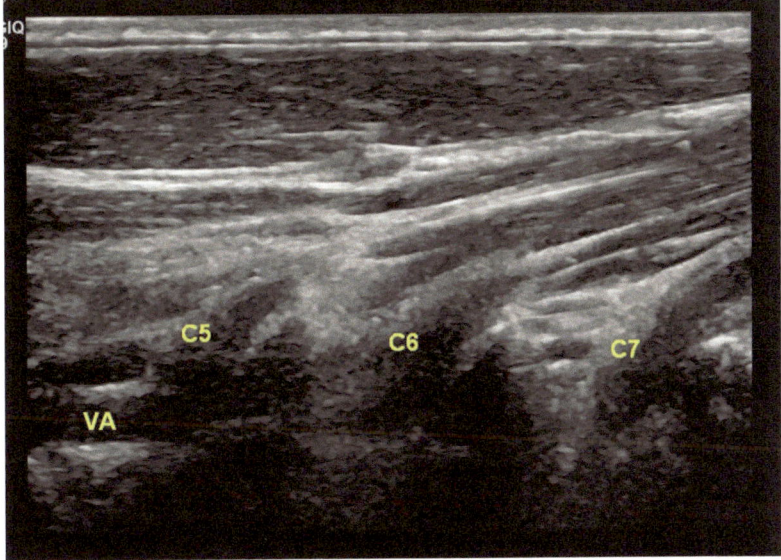

presents three circle-like hypoechoic structure; the superficial side is the rear edge of the sternocleidomastoid muscle.

3. Supraclavicular region: the head of the examinee is placed in the middle or slightly towards one side, and the upper arm is stretched outwards 20–30°. It is shown that at the lateral upper part of the cross section of the subclavian artery is the cross section of the brachial plexus in the supraclavicular region (see Fig. 2.9); on its deep part is the hyperechoic structure of the first rib, with an acoustic shadow behind.

4. Infraclavicular region: the probe is placed below the clavicle or 2 cm under the coracoid. On a parasagittal section, the cross sections of the axillary artery and axillary vein can be shown, while the three cords of the brachial plexus can be seen around blood vessels (see

Fig. 2.3 Normal longitudinal ultrasonogram of the C6 nerve root of the brachial plexus exiting the intervertebral foramen. Note: *VA* vertebral artery; C6 is the long axis of the brachial plexus; arrow 2 behind the vertebral artery indicates the nerve in the intervertebral foramen, and the hyperechoic structure indicated by the arrow beside C6 is the transverse process

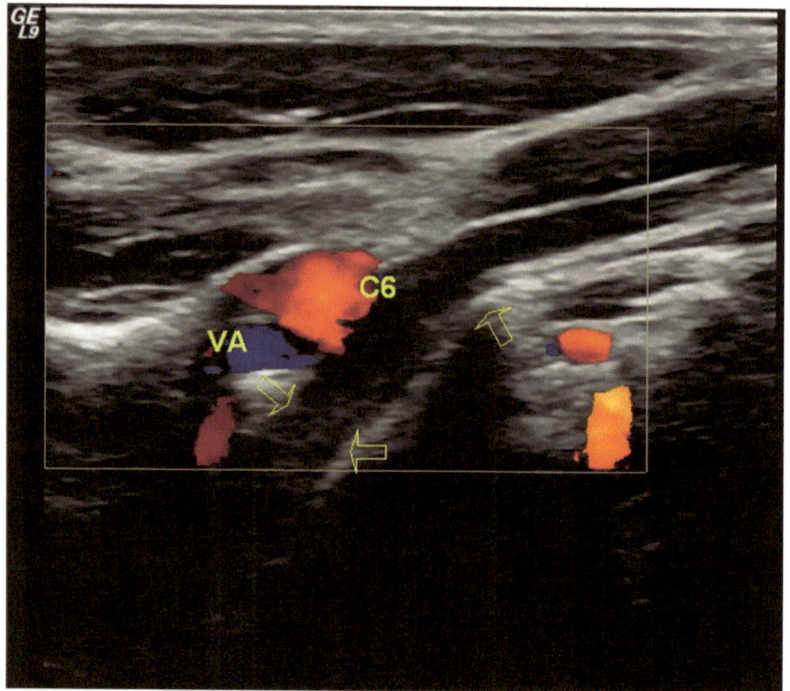

Fig. 2.4 Ultrasonogram of the posterior tubercle of the C7 nerve root. Note: *VA* vertebral artery, C5, C6 and C7 are the short axes of the nerve root of the brachial plexus, *PT* the posterior tubercle of C7

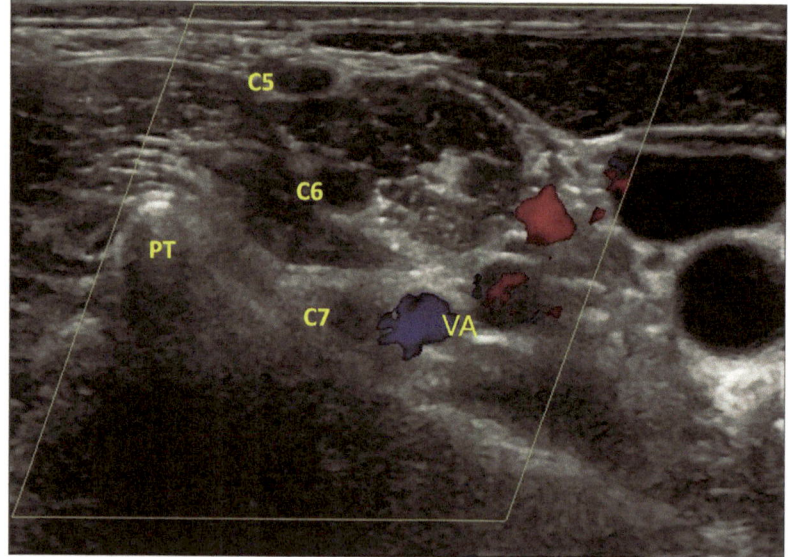

Figs. 2.10 and 2.11). The lateral cord is positioned outside the axillary artery, the medial cord is located between the axillary artery and the axillary vein, and the posterior cord is in the deep side of the axillary artery.

5. Axilla: the probe is placed in the axilla when the upper arms are stretch outwards 90° to locate the axillary artery and axillary vein. The radial nerve is located above the outside of the axillary artery, the median nerve is

Fig. 2.5 Ultrasonogram of the anterior and posterior tubercles of the C6 nerve root. Note: *AT* the anterior tubercle, C6 is the short axis of the nerve root of the brachial plexus, *PT* the posterior tubercle

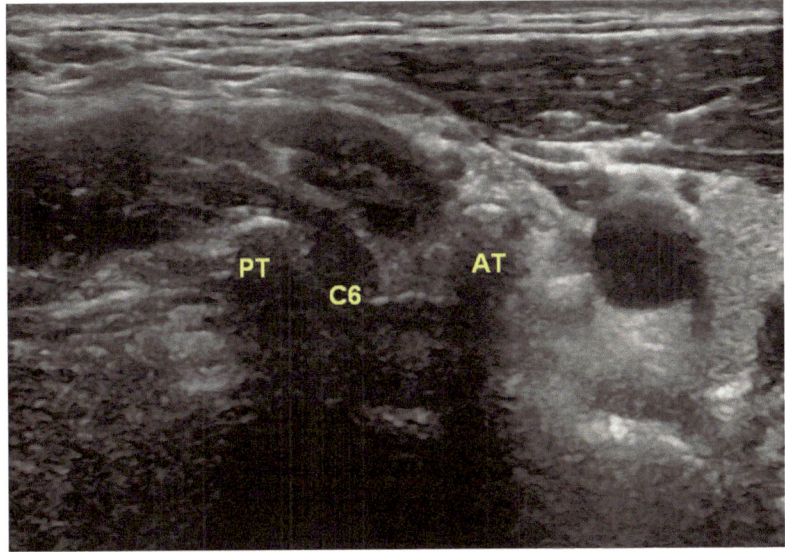

Fig. 2.6 Ultrasonogram of the anterior and posterior tubercles of the C5 nerve root. Note: *AT* the anterior tubercle, C5 is the short axis of the nerve root of the brachial plexus, *PT* the posterior tubercle

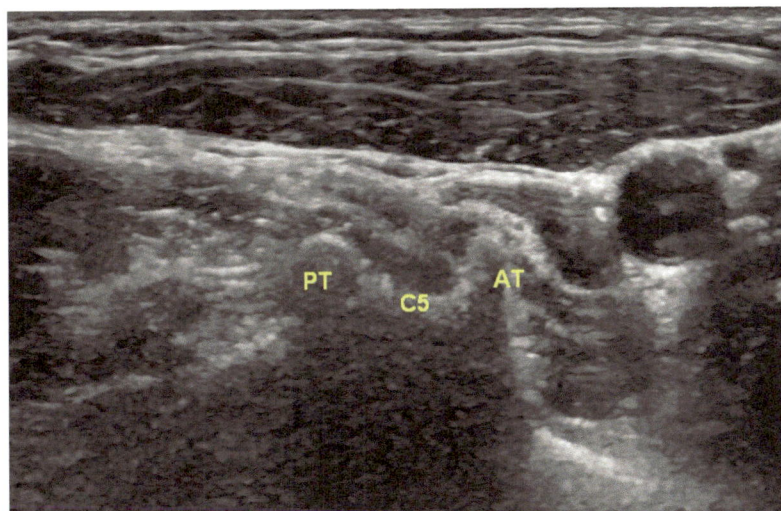

located between the axillary artery and axillary vein, and the ulnar nerve is behind the axillary artery. *The musculocutaneous nerve can also be shown in this view (see Fig. 2.12).*

ER 2.1 Dynamic image and explanation of the normal brachial plexus C6

ER 2.2 Dynamic image and explanation of normal brachial plexus scanning

ER 2.3 Dynamic image and explanation of normal C5 and C6 anterior and posterior tubercle scanning

2.2.2 Median Nerve

Methods for scanning the median nerve: the median nerve can be easily found on the transverse section in the middle of the forearm and upper arm, and can then be tracked horizontally

Fig. 2.7 Ultrasonogram of the anterior and posterior tubercles of the C4 nerve root. Note: *AT* the anterior tubercle, C4 is the short axis of the nerve root of the brachial plexus, *PT* the posterior tubercle

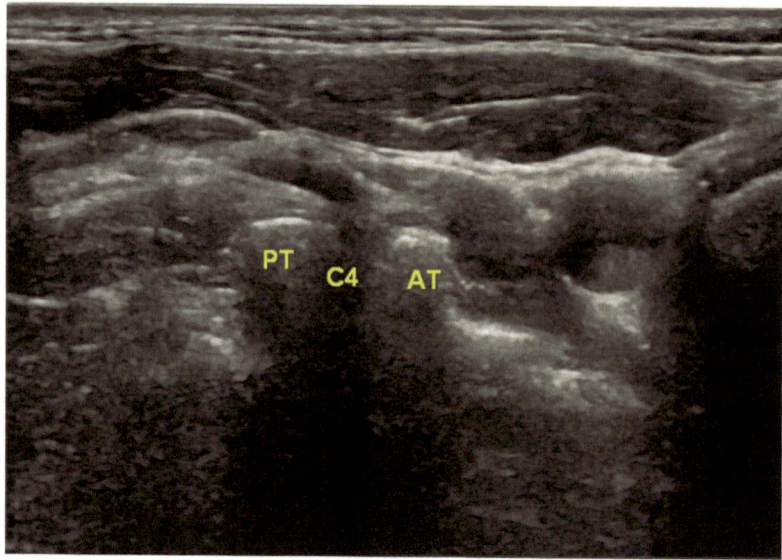

Fig. 2.8 Ultrasonogram of the interscalene section (superior, middle and inferior trunks) of the brachial plexus. Note: (**a**) shows the anterior scalene muscle; MS is the middle scalene muscle; the blue arrow indicates the superior trunk of the brachial plexus, the white arrow indicates the middle trunk of the brachial plexus, and the yellow arrow indicates the inferior trunk of the brachial plexus; (**b**) illustrates the scanning method of the brachial plexus at trunk level

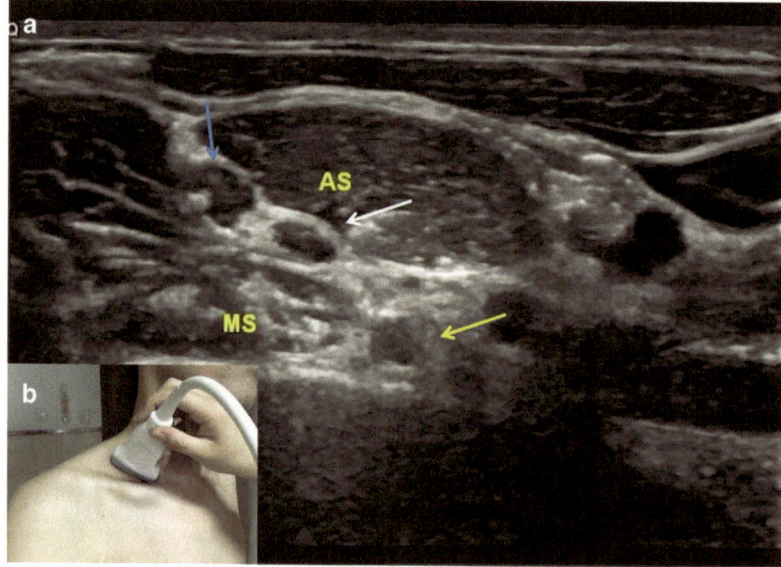

and vertically to the axilla and wrist for the longitudinal scanning of the nerves to observe their routes and the positions of entrapment (see Figs. 2.13 and 2.14) (Video 2.4).

ER 2.4 Dynamic image and explanation of normal forearm median nerve scanning

Anatomic variation in the median nerve includes the commonly seen bifid median nerve and persistent median artery. There is generally only one median nerve in the human body, but neural bifurcation is not rare and has an incidence rate of 3–19%. Bifurcation often occurs at the carpal canal level, but in some cases, the nerve is divided into two separate branches before entering the carpal canal. Alternatively, the nerve can also branch inside the carpal canal with no spacing between them (see Fig. 2.15). Sometimes, the bifid median nerve is also accompanied by the persistent median artery, and when this is observed by continuous

Fig. 2.9 Ultrasonogram of the supraclavicular region of the brachial plexus. Note: (**a**) SCA is subclavian artery, and BP refers to the cross section of the brachial plexus adjacent to the subclavian artery; (**b**) illustrates the scanning method of the brachial plexus at the clavicular fossa

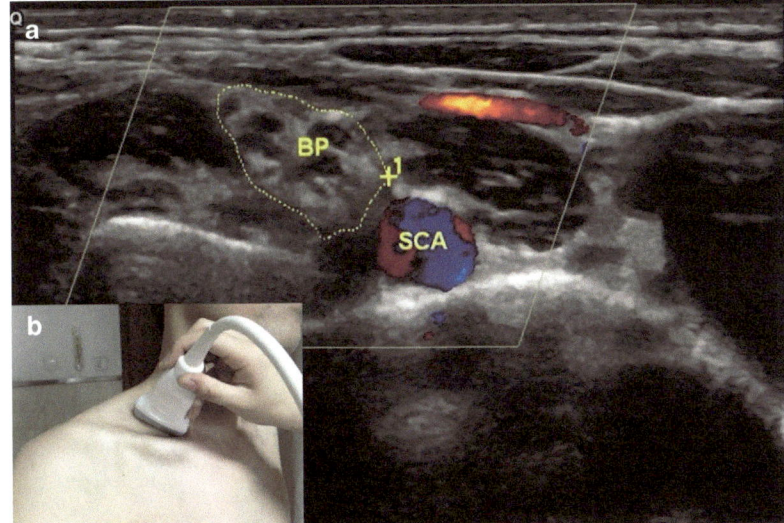

Fig. 2.10 Ultrasonogram of the brachial plexus at the level of the subclavian artery cord (long axis). Note: (**a**) SCA is subclavian artery, and the arrow indicates the long axis of the nerve cord level of the brachial plexus; (**b**) illustrates the scanning method of the nerve cord level of the brachial plexus

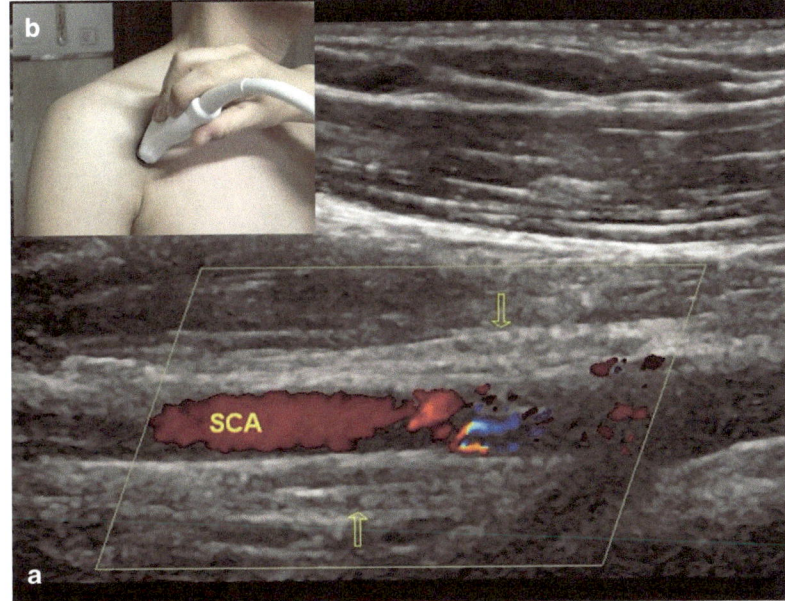

dynamic scanning, the persistent median artery is distinguished from the ulnar artery (the persistent median artery is usually coming from ulnar artery).

2.2.3   Radial Nerve

Methods for scanning the radial nerve: ultrasonic examination begins with horizontal and vertical transverse scanning at the humerus in close contact with radial nerve behind the upper arm. The nerve is then scanned on the longitudinal section—upwards between the start of the medial head and the lateral head of the musculus triceps brachii and downwards to the bifurcation of the superficial branch and deep branch at the lateral cubital fossa (see Figs. 2.16, 2.17, 2.18 and 2.19) (Videos 2.5, 2.6 and 2.7).

ER 2.5 Dynamic image and explanation of normal radial nerve scanning

Fig. 2.11 Ultrasonogram of the brachial plexus at the level of the subclavian artery (short axis). Note: the arrow points indicate the short axis of the nerve cord level; A is artery

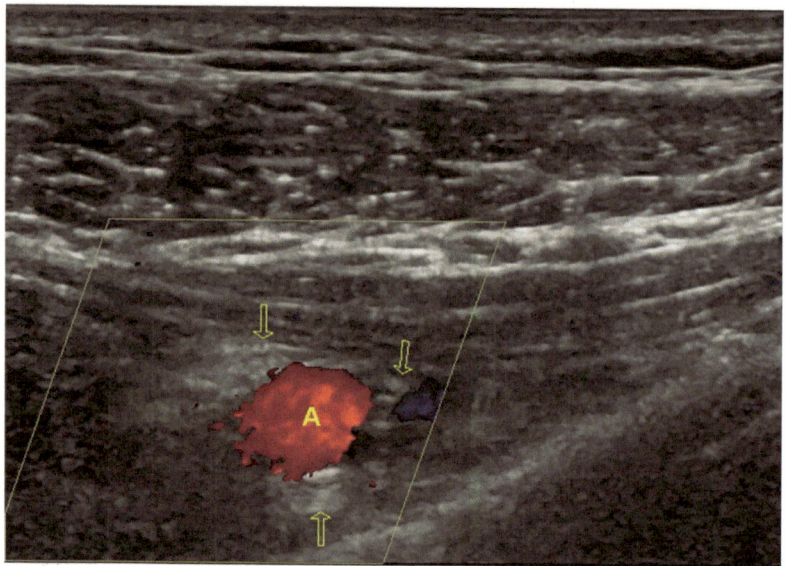

Fig. 2.12 Ultrasonogram of the brachial plexus at the level of the axilla (including the musculocutaneous nerve). Note: (**a**) MCN is the short axis of musculocutaneous nerve, MN is the short axis of median nerve, RN is the short axis of radial nerve and UN is the short axis of ulnar nerve; (**b**) is the diagram of how to scan the brachial plexus at the level of the axilla

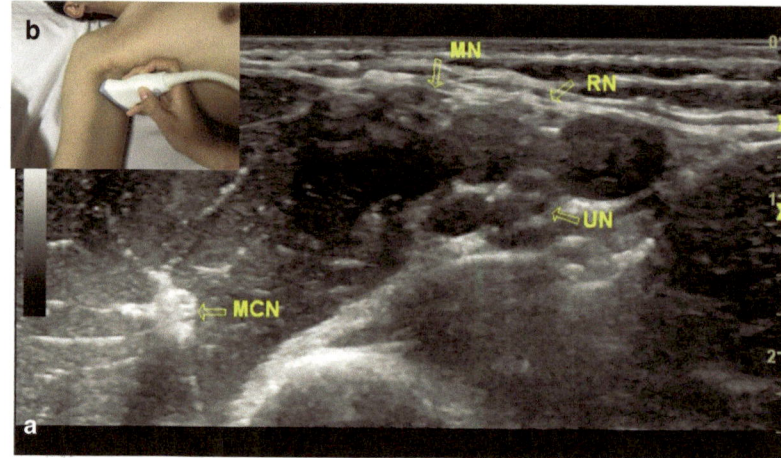

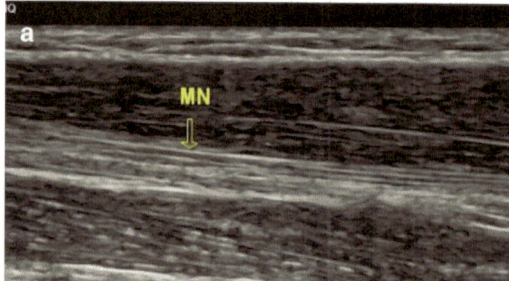
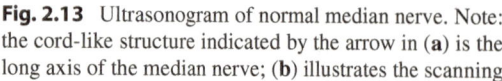
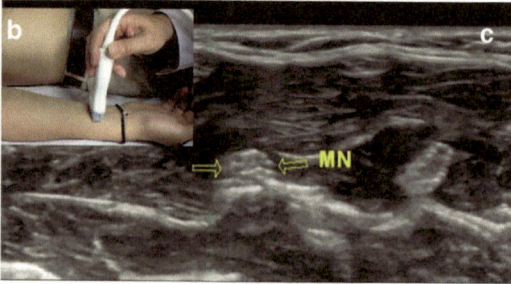

Fig. 2.13 Ultrasonogram of normal median nerve. Note: the cord-like structure indicated by the arrow in (**a**) is the long axis of the median nerve; (**b**) illustrates the scanning method of the short axis of the median nerve; the mesh-like structure indicated by the arrow in (**c**) is the short axis of the normal median nerve

Fig. 2.14 Ultrasonogram of cross sections of normal median nerve and ulnar nerve in the forearm. Note: *MN* median nerve, *UA* ulnar artery, *UN* ulnar nerve

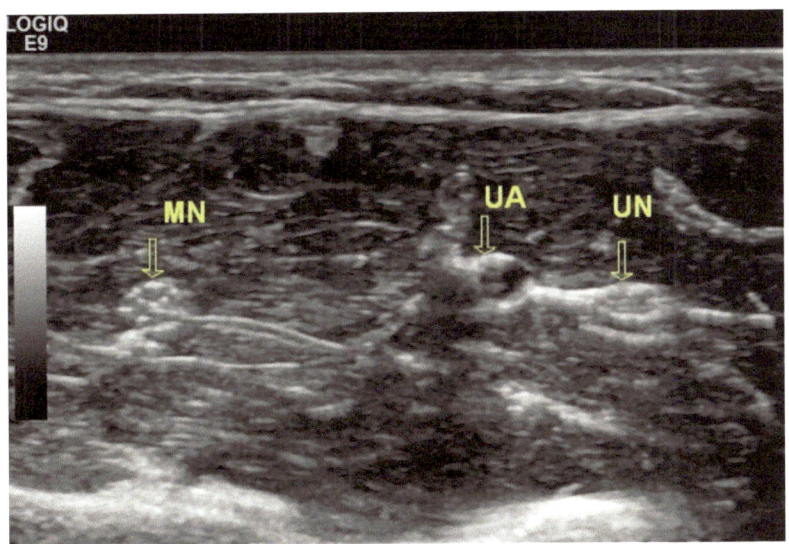

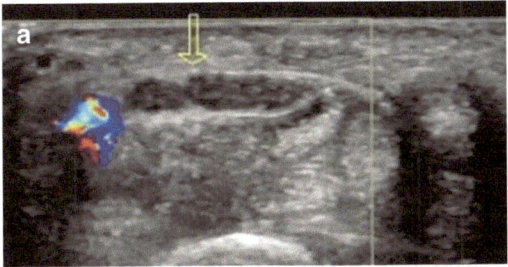

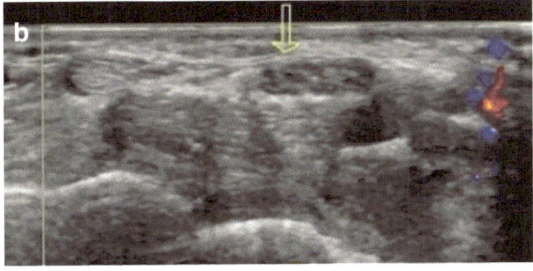

Fig. 2.15 Ultrasonogram of the anatomic variation (accessory median nerve) in the median nerve. Note: (**a**) is the diagram of accessory median nerve mutation; the arrow indicates the short axis of the accessory median nerve; (**b**) is a diagram of a normal median nerve; the arrow indicates the short axis of the median nerve

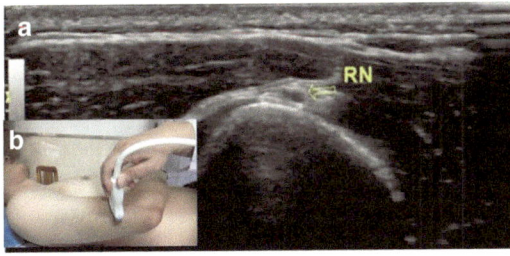

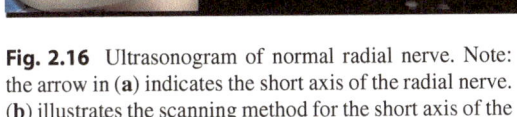

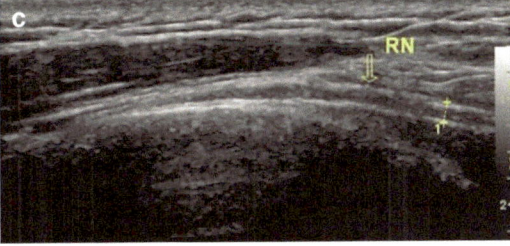

Fig. 2.16 Ultrasonogram of normal radial nerve. Note: the arrow in (**a**) indicates the short axis of the radial nerve. (**b**) illustrates the scanning method for the short axis of the radial nerve in the upper arm. The arrow in (**c**) indicates the long axis of the radial nerve. RN: radial nerve

Fig. 2.17 Ultrasonogram of cross sections of the superficial branch and deep branch of normal radial nerve. Note: the white arrow indicates the deep branch of the radial nerve, and the yellow arrow indicates the superficial branch of the radial nerve

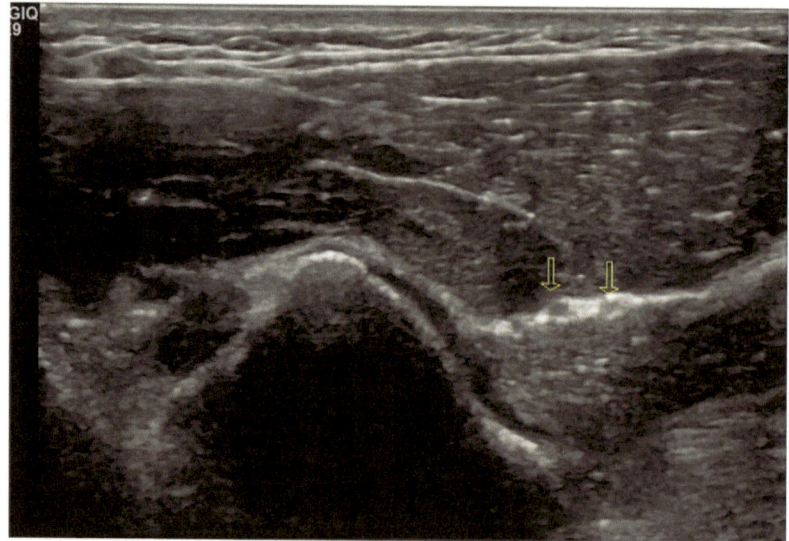

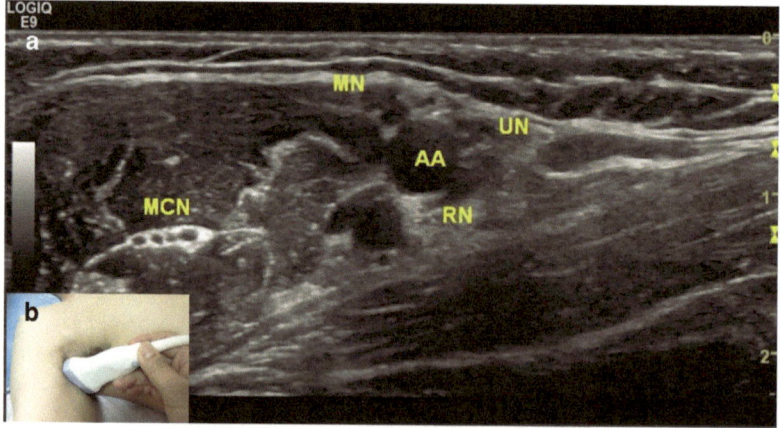

Fig. 2.18 Ultrasonogram of the short axis of a normal musculocutaneous nerve. Note: In (**a**) MCN means musculocutaneous nerve, MN means the short axis of the median nerve, RN is the short axis of the radial nerve, UN is the short axis of the ulnar nerve and AA is axillary artery; (**b**) illustrates the scanning of the musculocutaneous nerve at the level of the axilla in the upper arm

Fig. 2.19 Ultrasonogram of the long axis of normal musculocutaneous nerve. Note: the arrow points to the long axis of the musculocutaneous nerve

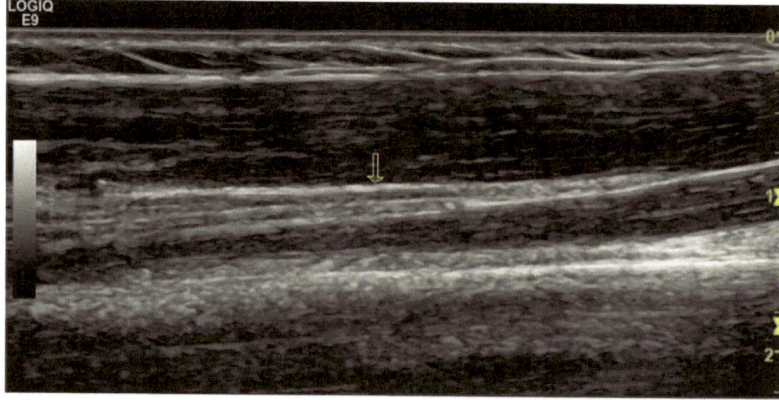

ER 2.6 Dynamic image and explanation of normal musculocutaneous nerve scanning

ER 2.7 Dynamic image and explanation of normal interosseous dorsal nerve scanning

2.2.4 Ulnar Nerve

Methods for scanning the ulnar nerve: the ultrasonic examination can begin with upward or downward tracking scanning from the ulnar nerve behind the elbow—the short-axis transverse section is scanned before examining the long-axis longitudinal section. The ulnar nerve behind the elbow is located in the ulnar nerve groove between the epicondylus extensorius and the olecranon. The ulnar nerve in the forearm is located between the ulnar flexor of the wrist and the flexor digitorum profundus, and the lower part of the ulnar nerve is located in the forearm where it runs along the ulnar artery, which can be regarded as ultrasonic location landmarks [7] (see Figs. 2.20, 2.21 and 2.22) (Video 2.8).

ER 2.8 Dynamic image and explanation of normal ulnar nerve scanning

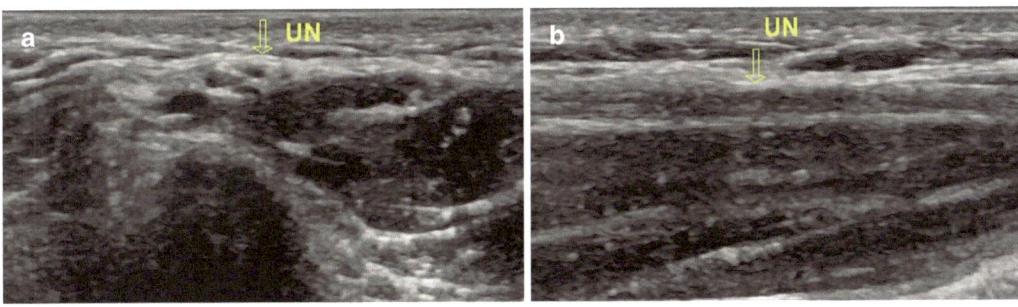

Fig. 2.20 Ultrasonogram of normal ulnar nerve. Note: *UN* ulnar nerve, the arrows indicate the short (**a**) and long axes (**b**) of normal ulnar nerve

Fig. 2.21 Ultrasonogram of the short axis of normal digital nerve. Note: N is digital nerve, A is digital artery. The white arrow indicates the short axis of the digital nerve and the yellow arrow indicates the short axis of the digital artery

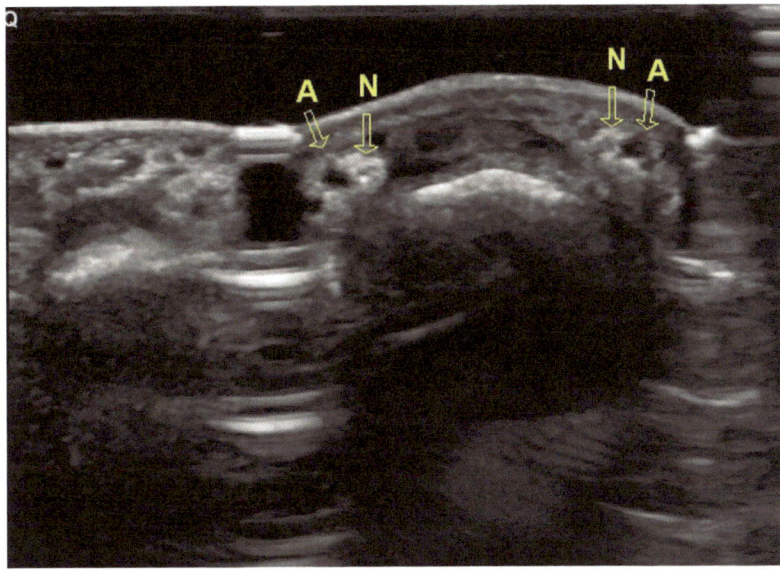

Fig. 2.22 Ultrasonogram of the long axis of normal digital nerve. Note: N indicates the digital nerve, and the white arrow indicates the long axis of the digital nerve; A indicates the digital artery and the yellow arrow indicates the long axis of the digital artery

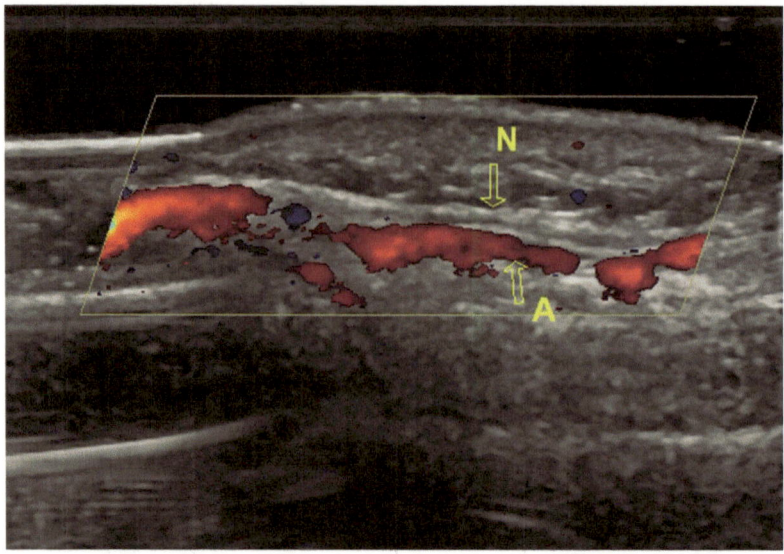

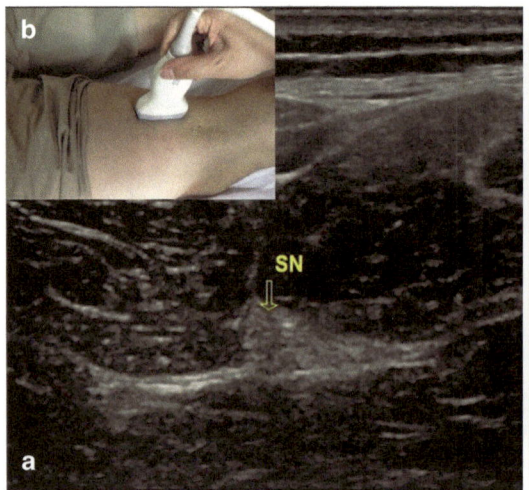

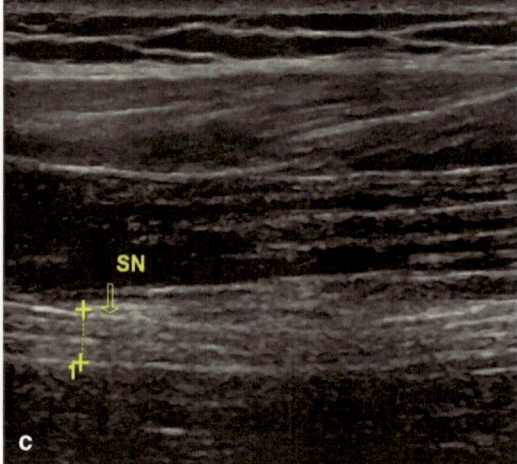

Fig. 2.23 Ultrasonogram of the short and long axes of normal sciatic nerve. Note: *SN* sciatic nerve. In (**a**) the arrow indicates the short axis of the sciatic nerve, (**b**) illustrates the scanning of the long axis of the sciatic nerve in the lower limbs, and in (**c**), the arrow indicates the long axis of the sciatic nerve

2.2.5 Sciatic Nerve, Tibial Nerve and Common Peroneal Nerve

Methods for scanning sciatic nerve, tibial nerve and common peroneal nerve: ultrasonic examination starts below the popliteal space of the lower limbs for the horizontal and vertical scanning of the transverse section. Then, the sciatic nerve can be seen upwards beside the popliteal artery and popliteal vein, and at this point, the ultrasonogram shows the mesh structure on the transverse section of the sciatic nerve (see Fig. 2.23 and Video 2.9). The sciatic nerve that runs downwards branches into the tibial and common peroneal nerves. The tibial nerve is located beside the popliteal artery and popliteal vein, with its long axis running along the tibial artery (see Fig. 2.24), while the common peroneal nerve runs downwards from the lateral side and bypasses the

Fig. 2.24 Ultrasonogram of the long axis of normal common peroneal nerve. Note: the arrow indicates the long axis of the common peroneal nerve

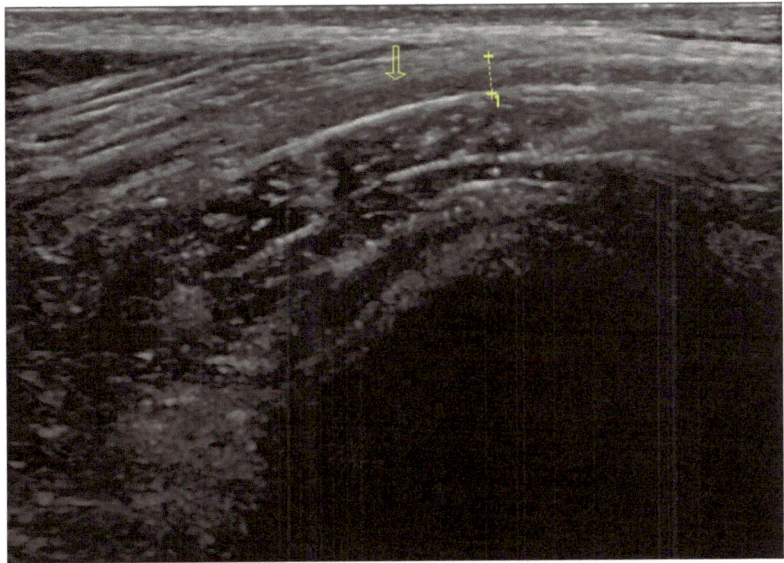

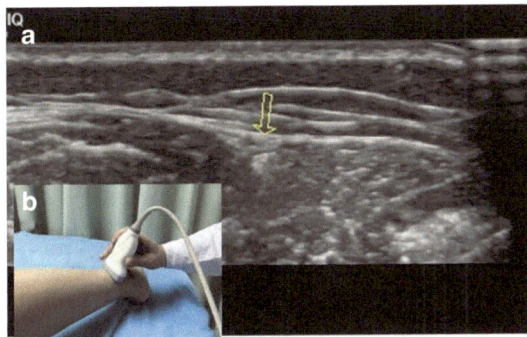

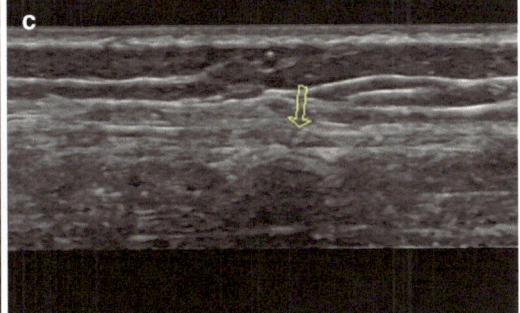

Fig. 2.25 Ultrasonogram of normal superficial peroneal nerve. Note: the arrow in (**a**) is pointing to the short axis of the superficial peroneal nerve and (**b**) illustrates the scanning of normal superficial peroneal nerve. The arrow in (**c**) is pointing to the long axis of the superficial peroneal nerve

fibular head, under which it is divided into the superficial peroneal nerve and the deep peroneal nerve (see Figs. 2.25 and 2.26). The former is located between the extensor digitorum longus, peroneus longus and short peroneal, while the latter runs downwards along with the anterior tibial artery.

Mutation of the sciatic nerve route: below the lower edge of the piriformis is the most typical position by which the sciatic nerve exits the pelvis, but it can also start from the upper edge of the piriformis. Most sciatic nerves generally branch into the tibial nerve and peroneal nerve at the popliteal space or at its proximal end, but some may branch at higher positions (Video 2.10).

ER 2.9 Dynamic image and explanation of normal sciatic nerve root scanning

ER 2.10 Dynamic image and explanation of normal sciatic nerve, tibial nerve and common peroneal nerve scanning

2.2.6   Femoral Nerve and Saphenous Nerve

Methods for scanning the femoral nerve and saphenous nerve: the probe starts scanning from the anterior superior iliac spine and then slides to the symphysis pubis along the inguinal

Fig. 2.26 Ultrasonogram of normal tibial nerve. Note: the yellow arrow indicates the popliteal artery and at the Vernier calliper is the long axis of the posterior tibial nerve

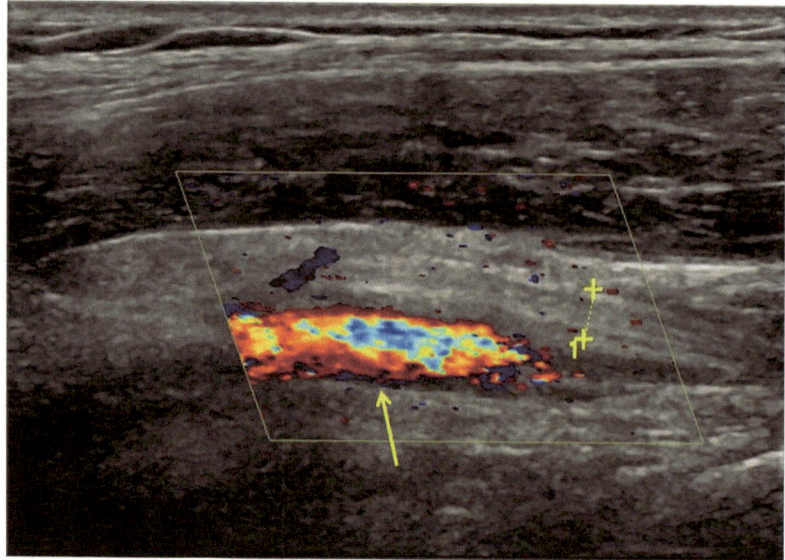

Fig. 2.27 Ultrasonogram of the long axis of normal femoral nerve. Note: the yellow arrow indicates the long axis of the femoral nerve; A indicates femoral artery

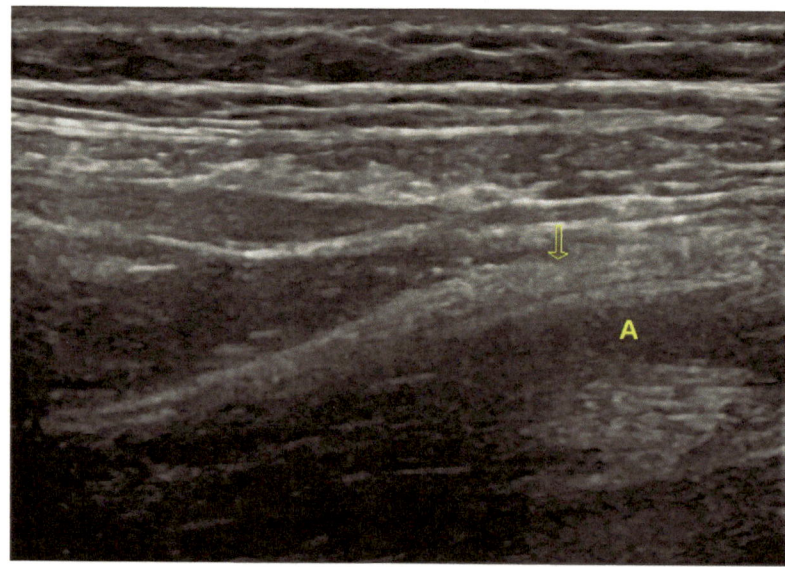

ligament. The femoral nerve is found between the iliopsoas and the femoral artery. Then, the probe is moved vertically downwards along the thigh until it reaches position at 1/3 of the front and inner side of the thigh. At this moment, the adductor canal, which is the hyperechoic triangular structure at the front and slightly inner side of the thighbone, can be seen. The femoral nerve in the shallow part and the femoral vein in the deep part can be seen; the mesh struc-

ture is the saphenous nerve, which is located in front of and outside the femoral nerve (see Figs. 2.27, 2.28 and 2.29) (Videos 2.11 and 2.12).

ER 2.11 Dynamic image and explanation of normal femoral nerve scanning

ER 2.12 Dynamic image and explanation of normal saphenous nerve scanning

Fig. 2.28 Ultrasonogram of the short axis of normal femoral nerve. Note: the yellow arrow indicates the short axis of the femoral nerve; A indicates femoral artery

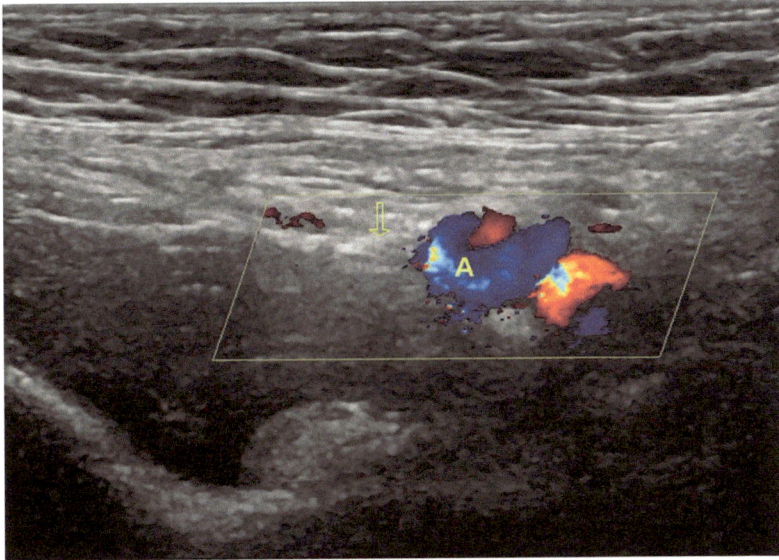

Fig. 2.29 Ultrasonogram of the short axis of normal saphenous nerve. Note: (**a**) the yellow arrow indicates the short axis of the saphenous nerve; the asterisk indicates the artery; (**b**) illustrates the scanning of normal saphenous nerve

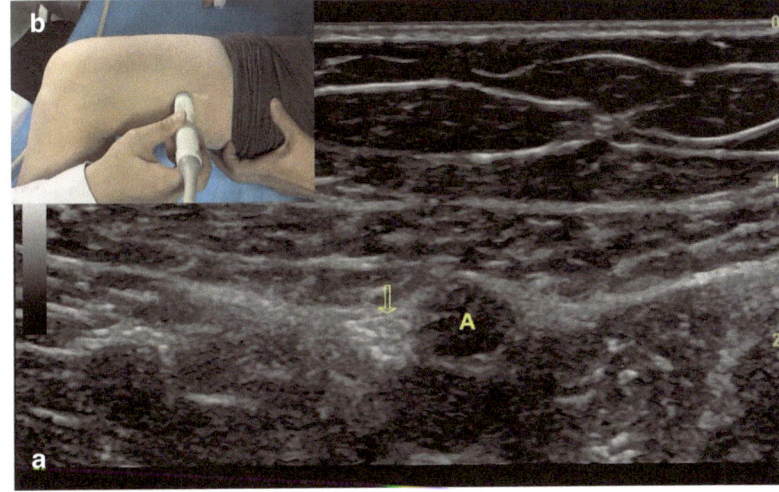

2.3   Measuring Methods and Normal Values

The measurement of peripheral nerves mainly includes the diameter and cross-sectional area. For the measurement of nerve diameter, an ultrasound beam should be vertical to the nerve long-axis or short-axis section while measuring the vertical diameter or the transverse diameter between the epineurium and the contralateral epineurium (see Fig. 2.30) (see Tables 2.1 and 2.2 for normal peripheral nerve diameters as reference values). To measure the cross-sectional area of the nerve, the trace description method should be used as an ultrasound beam is vertical to the short-axis section for scanning (see Fig. 2.31).

Pay heed to adjustment of the probe to ensure that the ultrasound beam is vertical to the nerve for accurate measurement.

Fig. 2.30 Ultrasonogram of the long-axis measurement of normal median nerve. Note: the Vernier calliper shows the long-axis measurement of the median nerve

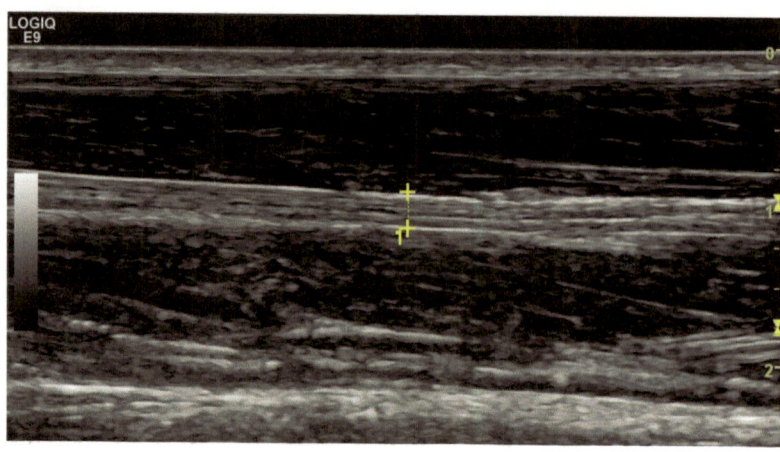

Table 2.1 Normal reference values of bilateral brachial plexus diameter in adults (mm)

Name	C5	C6	C7	C8
Left brachial plexus	3.25 ± 0.34	3.36 ± 0.30	3.55 ± 0.29	3.51 ± 0.27
Right brachial plexus	3.20 ± 0.26	3.38 ± 0.28	3.57 ± 0.24	3.54 ± 0.21

Table 2.2 Normal reference values of the primary peripheral nerves in the upper and lower limbs in adults

	Nerve diameter (mm)		Cross-sectional area of nerve (mm^2)	
	Left	Right	Left	Right
Median nerve	2.31 ± 0.26	2.33 ± 0.27	7.45 ± 1.91	7.31 ± 1.95
Ulnar nerve	2.23 ± 0.37	2.20 ± 0.33	6.75 ± 1.67	6.80 ± 1.65
Radial nerve	2.35 ± 0.28	2.33 ± 0.26	6.08 ± 1.45	6.10 ± 1.44
Sciatic nerve	5.36 ± 1.35	5.40 ± 1.46	50.01 ± 10.46	56.12 ± 10.22
Tibial nerve	3.48 ± 1.13	3.52 ± 1.10	43.21 ± 7.69	42.11 ± 7.56
Common peroneal nerve	2.82 ± 0.68	2.91 ± 0.71	13.92 ± 4.22	14.13 ± 4.53

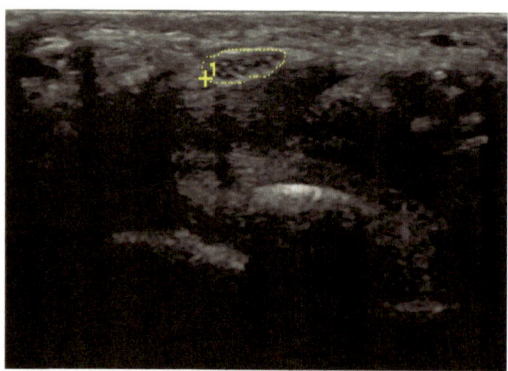

Fig. 2.31 Ultrasonogram of the short-axis cross-sectional area measurement of normal median nerve at the wrist. Note: the dashed line at the Vernier calliper is the short-axis cross-sectional area measurement of the median nerve

References

1. Wang J, Liu J. Musculoskeletal ultrasound. Beijing: Scientific and Technical Documentation Press; 2007.
2. Cui L. Atlas of peripheral nerve ultrasound. Beijing: Peking University Medical Press; 2004.
3. Wang Y. Fundamentals of musculoskeletal ultrasound. Beijing: Science Press; 2003.
4. Guo R. Musculoskeletal ultrasound. Beijing: People's Medical Publishing House; 2008.
5. Srivastava PK. High resolution ultrasound of brachial plexus. Ultrasound Med Biol. 2017;43(1):242.
6. Zhu YS, Mu NN, Zheng MJ, et al. High-resolution ultrasonography for the diagnosis of brachial plexus root lesions. Ultrasound Med Biol. 2014;40(7):1420–6.
7. Coraci D, Giovannini S, Imbimbo I, et al. Ulnar nerve dislocation at the elbow: the role of ultrasound. World Neurosurg. 2017;103:934–5.

Ultrasonography of Peripheral Nerve Abnormalities

3

Dingzhang Chen, Minjuan Zheng, Jing Wang, and Yunan Jia

3.1 Common Causes

3.1.1 Nerve Injury

Nerve swelling accompanied by a hypoechoic structure is a common occurrence in peripheral nerve entrapment syndrome and is also indicative of a sort of tumour-like hyperplasia after nerve injury. Nerve entrapment often occurs at the bone fibre canals or tunnels, such as the median nerve in the carpal canal, the ulnar nerve in the cubital tunnel, the common peroneal nerve in the fibular canal at the fibular head and the tibial nerve in the tarsal tunnel. The nerve generally presents a narrow radial line at the entrapment where the proximal and/or distal end is swollen, which is seen along with hypoechoic changes and the absence of a mesh or layer structure.

Fibrous tumour-like hyperplasia after nerve injury often presents as swelling of the local nerve, and even a tumour-like swelling can be observed. These injuries can be caused either by direct damage, such as iatrogenic incised wounds, or by chronic lesions, such as Morton's neuroma.

For research on an animal injury model, the author established a chronic sciatic nerve entrapment model designed by Mackinnon to observe the changes in ultrasonoscopy, nerve electrophysiology and pathology by comparison with the control group. During that study, it was found that the epineurium on the long axis section of the sciatic nerve in the control group presents a parallel stripe-like isoechoic structure, with a stronger linear beam echoic structure inside. The transverse section had a round or oval ring-like echoic structure, with scattered echogenic dots inside. The results of the ultrasonic examination on sciatic nerve entrapment for each group are discussed below. For the group with entrapment for 2 weeks, at the entrapment and at both ends of the sciatic nerve, the nerve was slightly thickened. Its inner echo with a poor linear continuity was obviously reduced, but its epineurium had tidy edges and was not thickened, and the inner echo of the compressed nerve was obviously decreased. For the group with entrapment for 4 weeks, at the entrapment and at both ends of the sciatic nerve, the nerve was obviously thickened. Its inside was hypoechoic and disordered with an inhomogeneous linear echo, and its epineurium had untidy edges that were slightly thickened. For the group with entrapment for 6–8 weeks, at the entrapment and at both ends, the sciatic nerve diameter was obviously thicker, and a portion of it had tumour-like changes. Its inner echo was shown as a disor-

Supplementary Information The online version contains supplementary material available at https://doi.org/10.1007/978-981-15-2704-3_3.

D. Chen (✉) · M. Zheng · J. Wang · Y. Jia
Department of Ultrasound, Xijing Hospital,
Fourth Military Medical University,
Xi'an, Shaanxi, China

dered, inhomogeneous linear continuity that was hypoechoic, and its epineurium had untidy edges that were slightly thickened.

The typical ultrasonogram of the longitudinal section of the sciatic nerve in the group with entrapment after 6 weeks is shown in Fig. 3.1. The silicone tube-wrapped nerve is shown as a hyperechoic linear structure, and the nerve echogenicity is reduced in the entrapment area. After removal of the silicone tube, the anatomical specimens showed that the nerve was thin at the entrapment level and that its epineurium at both ends had slight hyperaemia and presented with slight, tumour-like changes. Moreover, the ultrasonogram is very sensitive to tissue oedema and its corresponding volume changes, and since the nerve's axoplasmic flow at the entrapment is blocked, the water content of the tissue is increased (see Figs. 3.2 and 3.3). These research results suggest that high-frequency ultrasound can show changes in the different phases of rabbit sciatic nerve injury in real time, while the extent of peripheral nerve injury can be observed dynamically and accurately, which offers a reference for clinical diagnosis, treatment and prognosis.

3.1.2 Neurological Space-Occupying Lesion

Neurological space-occupying lesion includes neurogenic tumours and traumatic neuromas.

Neurogenic tumours, which often develop in the peripheral main trunk, subcutaneous or superficial muscle groups, are easily discernible and diagnosed. Doctors who are inexperienced in identifying these masses without obvious clinical symptoms often misdiagnose such masses as lymph glands, haematomas, myofibromas or haemangiomas, and they remove them along with surrounding nerves. Sometimes, the nerves are damaged, which leads to iatrogenic nerve impairment. Common tumours mainly include schwannoma and neurofibroma.

Traumatic neuroma, one of the most common complications of peripheral nerve injury, forms primarily because of the regeneration or even the reversed overlap of fractured nerve fibres due to squeezing, incision, avulsion or ischaemia. This leads to enlargement of the local nerve (shuttle shaped) or tumour-like changes at the fracture.

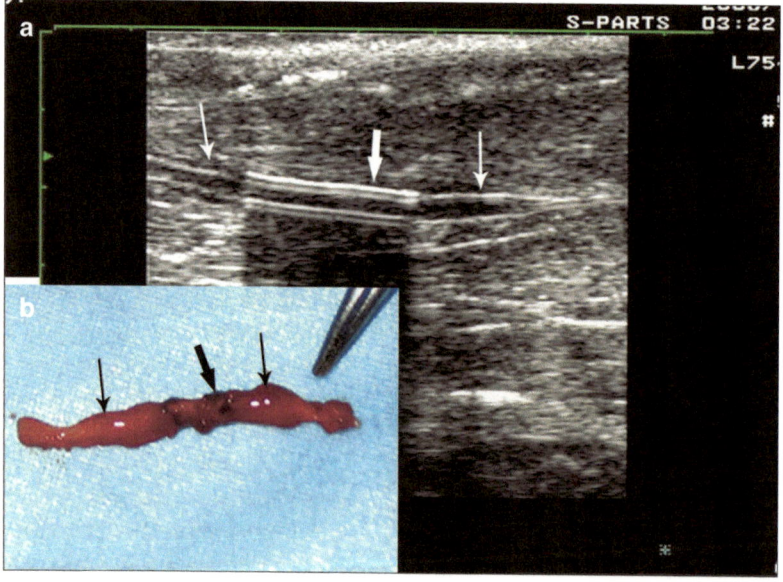

Fig. 3.1 Ultrasonogram and specimen diagram of rabbit sciatic nerve injury. Note: (**a**) Ultrasonogram of the longitudinal section of sciatic nerve. The slim arrow indicates the enlarged sciatic nerve at both ends of the entrapment, with a disordered linear echo, and an obviously thickened epineurium. The silicone tube is wrapped by a hyper-echoic linear structure (bold arrow), while the nerve in the entrapment area was hypoechoic. (**b**) The anatomical sample after the silicone tube was removed; the nerve was thin at the entrapment level (bold arrow), and the nerve at both ends shows slight hyperaemia and slight tumour-like changes (slim arrow)

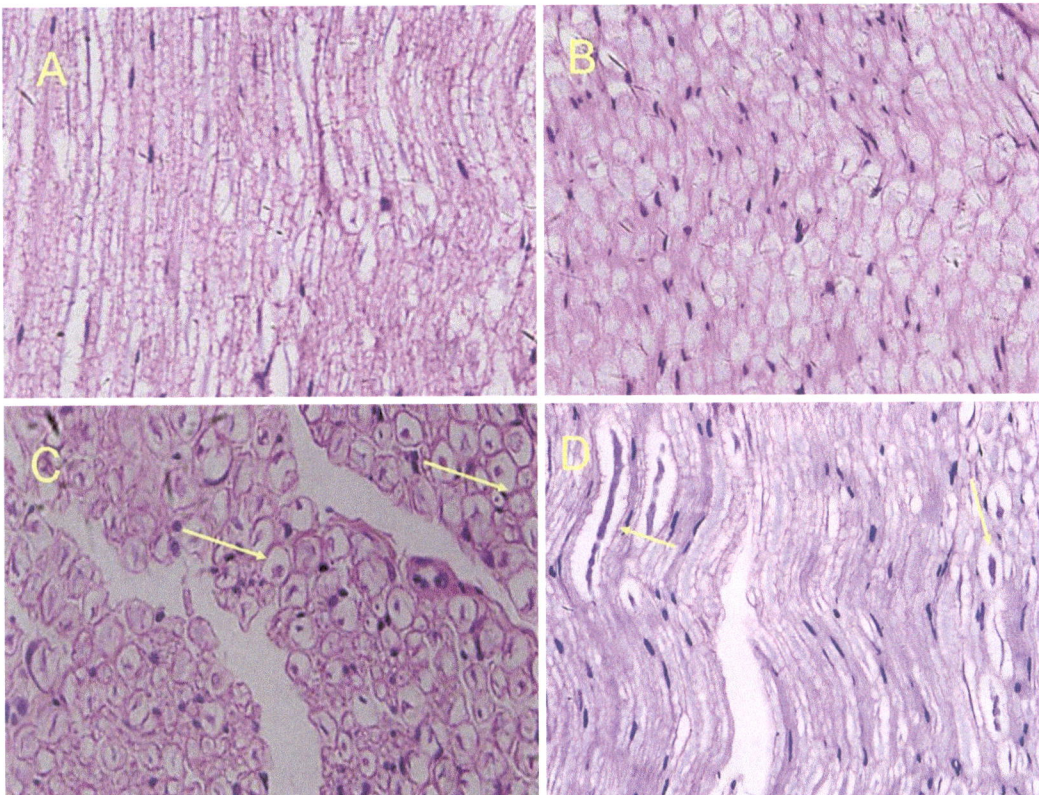

Fig. 3.2 Pathology of rabbit sciatic nerve entrapment. Note: (**a, b**) are the optical microscopy images of the longitudinal and transverse sections of normal rabbit sciatic nerve; (**c**) is the optical micrograph of the transverse section from the group that experienced entrapment for 2 weeks; an obviously swollen myelin sheath and an increased gap between the sheath and the axon are shown (arrow); (**d**) is the group that experienced entrapment for 8 weeks; obviously twisted axons and a broken myelin sheath are shown (HE ×40)

According to the existence of the nerve continuity, the traumatic neuroma can be divided into incomplete traumatic neuroma and completely disconnected neuroma.

3.2 Common Diseases and Relevant Ultrasonograms

3.2.1 Nerve Entrapment and Traumatic Lesions

Peripheral nerve entrapment syndrome refers to a special kind of peripheral nerve injury caused by mechanical compression of the nerve by the surrounding narrow and solid tissues contacting some section or some point of a peripheral nerve. Entrapment is the most common condition in hand surgery. Patients' clinical symptoms in the upper limbs mainly include discomfort in the neck and shoulders, numb hands and weak upper limbs, as well as amyotrophy of the hands and upper limbs, while symptoms in the lower limbs mainly include a painful, uncomfortable, weak waist and numb feet.

According to peripheral nerve anatomy, entrapment often occurs at the sheathing canal, fractures, rings or holes and is related to the dissected structure's volume, including content and neural entrapment resistance. Peripheral nerve entrapment syndrome is generally triggered by many factors, or a combination of factors, and of these, anatomical factors are the most common.

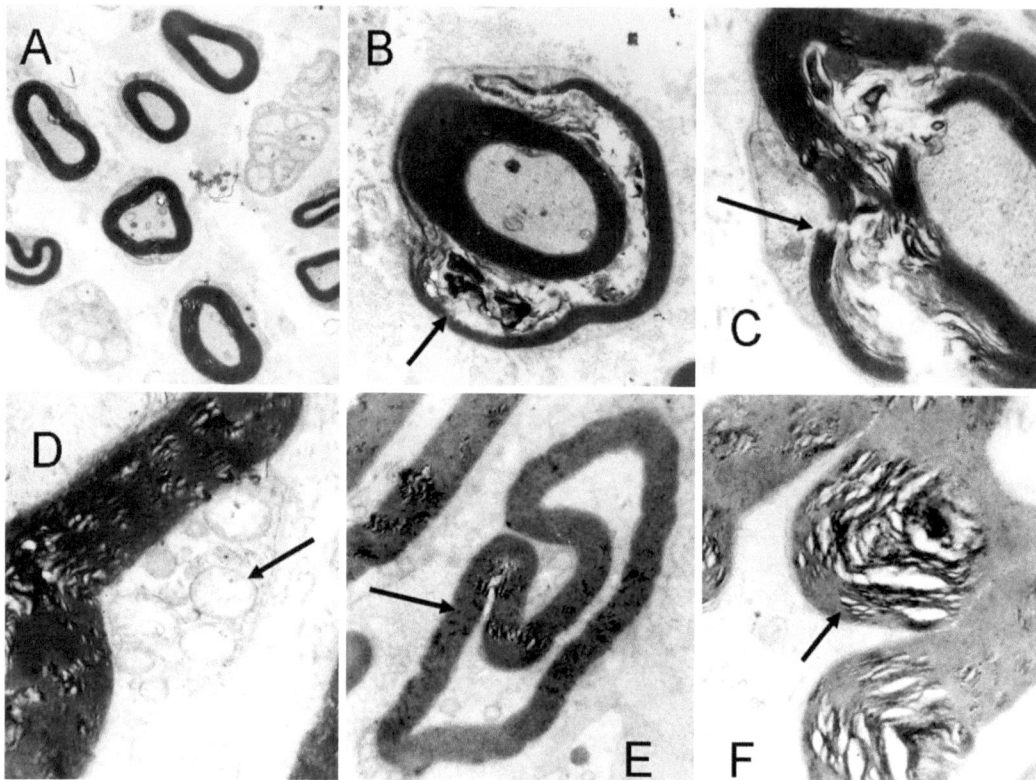

Fig. 3.3 Electron microscopy of rabbit sciatic nerve entrapment. Note: (**a**) normal myelin sheath from a control animal (×4000); (**b**) entrapment for 2 weeks; the arrow indicates the obviously separated myelin sheath slab (×7500); (**c**) entrapment for 2 weeks; the arrow indicates the deformed myelin sheath, with its slab separated and broken (×15,000); (**d**) entrapment for 4 weeks; the arrow indicates mitochondrial swelling and vesiculation in Schwann cells (×15,000); (**e**) entrapment for 8 weeks; the arrow indicates the obviously deformed myelin sheath (×12,000); (**f**) entrapment for 8 weeks; the arrow indicates the separated and structurally disordered slab inside the myelin sheath (×15,000)

This disease is mostly associated with repetitive movements. For example, overuse of the fingers to clamp objects may cause digital nerve entrapment; carpal tunnel syndrome is related to excessive movements of the fingers (such as hand kitting), so that the synovial membrane in the carpal tunnel becomes oedematous and thus compresses the median nerve; cubital tunnel syndrome is related to excessive movements of elbow joints.

3.2.1.1 Brachial Plexus Injury

Preganglionic injury of the brachial plexus often occurs at the root of the brachial plexus, where the nerve gradually becomes thin, with the disruption or disappearance of nerve continuity (Figs. 3.4 and 3.5), while the nerve at the distal end outside the intervertebral foramen becomes enlarged, and often a cyst appears beside the neural canal due to leakage of cerebrospinal fluid [1, 2] (Video 3.1).

ER 3.1 Dynamic image and explanation of brachial plexus preganglionic injury

Unlike the normal-side of the brachial plexus, the transverse section of the early brachial plexus postganglionic injury is clearly swollen, enlarged, and hypoechoic and demonstrates adhesion to surrounding tissues; the neural beam echo on the longitudinal section has disappeared and is distorted [3, 4] (see Figs. 3.6 and 3.7) (Videos 3.2 and 3.3).

Fig. 3.4 Ultrasonogram of preganglionic root avulsion of the brachial plexus. Note: (**a**) shows the discontinuity of the C6 and C7 nerve roots; M indicates formation of tumour-like changes of nerve root avulsion, and the yellow arrow indicates nerve root avulsion; (**b**) is the surgical procedure of preganglionic root avulsion of the brachial plexus

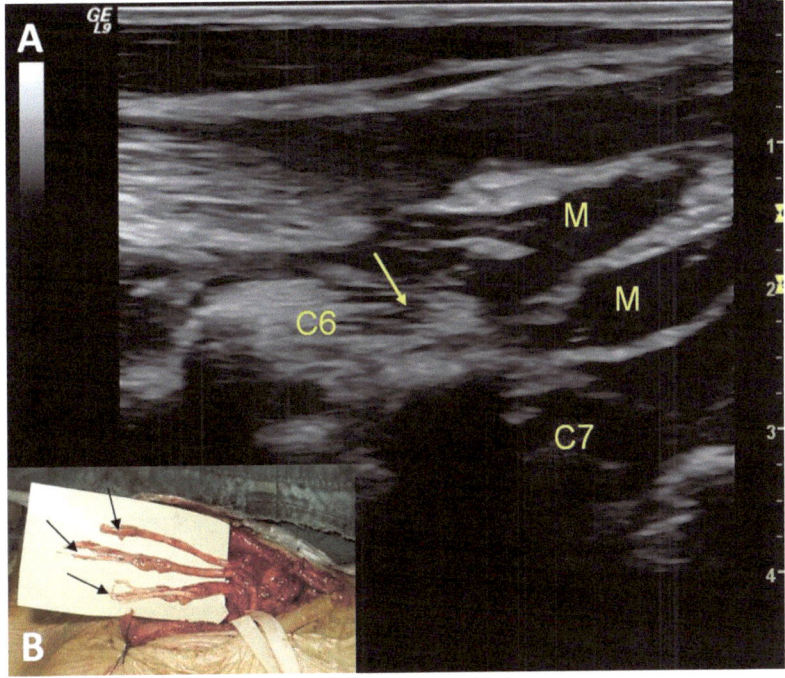

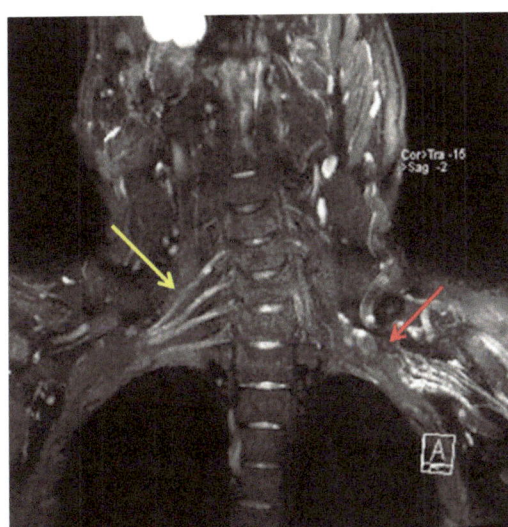

Fig. 3.5 MRI of root avulsion of the brachial plexus. Note: the yellow arrow indicates the normal brachial plexus, while the red arrow indicates root avulsion of the brachial plexus on the other side

ER 3.2 Dynamic image and explanation of brachial plexus postganglionic superior trunk injury

ER 3.3 Dynamic image and explanation of brachial plexus postganglionic injury

3.2.1.2 Median Nerve Injury

Median nerve injury often occurs at the wrists and leads to functional impairment of the hands due to a twisted or partly fractured median nerve by incised wounds. The ultrasonogram shows that the nerve continuity is disrupted completely or partially (see Fig. 3.8). The nerve is clearly thickened around the injury and has a hypoechoic structure, and a neuroma may form at both ends of the injured nerve (see Fig. 3.9).

Carpal tunnel syndrome is caused by compression of the median nerve as it passes through the carpal tunnel, which is a common cause of hand numbness and pain (the symptoms lessen at night), and results from increased pressure inside the carpal tunnel. The two main reasons are: (1) decreased carpal tunnel volume (the cross-sectional area of the carpal tunnel is reduced), which may be related to degenerative changes in the bones and joints at the wrists and ligament ossification of the carpus. (2) The increased contents in the carpal tunnel such as hyperplasia, aseptic inflammation and fibrosis of the synovial membrane in the carpal tunnel lead to an increase of the contents inside, which thus causes increased pressure in the carpal tunnel [5]. All the

Fig. 3.6 Ultrasonogram of brachial plexus postganglionic superior trunk injury. Note: C5 and C6 exit the nerve root; the arrow indicates the thickened C5 and C6 nerves with oedema at their distal ends

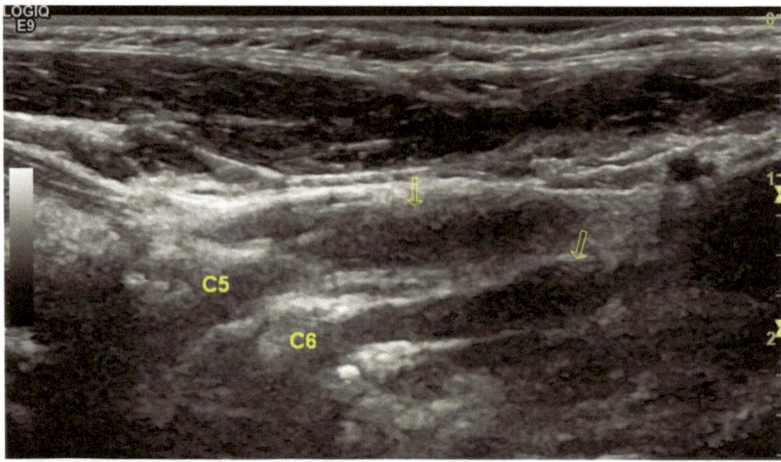

Fig. 3.7 Ultrasonogram of brachial plexus postganglionic nerve oedema. Note: C5, C6, C7, C8 of the brachial plexus network are thickened with oedema; the yellow arrow indicates the vertebral artery

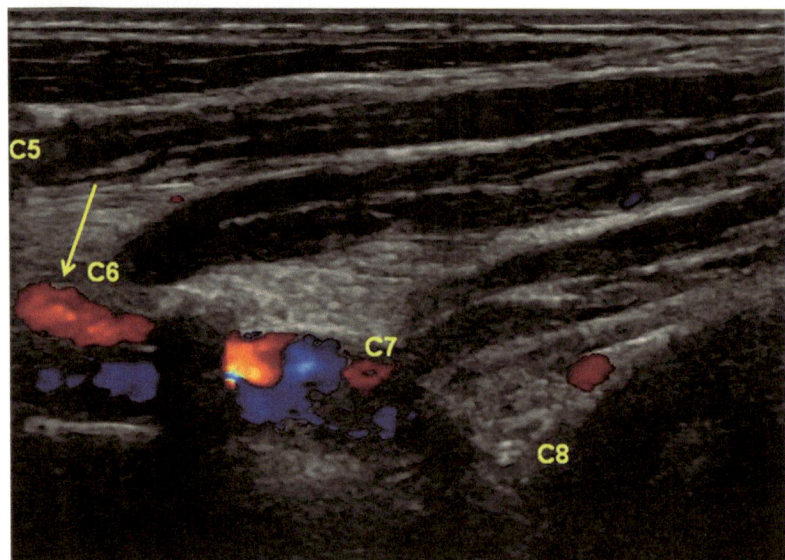

factors mentioned above are related to overuse of the wrist. In general, median nerve entrapment often occurs under the transverse carpal ligament.

Diagnosis: (1) the three and a half fingers innervated by the radial nerve have numbness and pain. Such symptoms become more severe at night, and the patient may sometimes suddenly awaken; the symptoms then gradually disappear when shaking or rubbing the hands. (2) In severe cases, the thenar muscle atrophies, thus limiting the opposing functions of the thumbs. (3) Electrophysiological examination: fibrillation potential occurs at the thenar muscle, and sensation in the median nerve and

the conduction velocity of the motor nerve are decreased. (4) Ultrasound shows that the median nerve at the carpal canal is enlarged at the proximal end of the entrapment where the nerve becomes thin and has a hypoechoic structure (Fig. 3.10).

3.2.1.3 Ulnar Nerve Injury

Cubital tunnel syndrome is a syndrome of ulnar nerve entrapment at the elbows. The cubital tunnel is also a bone fibre tube through which the ulnar nerve runs and often encounters entrapment. The common causes include: (1) the malunion and cubitus valgus after elbow

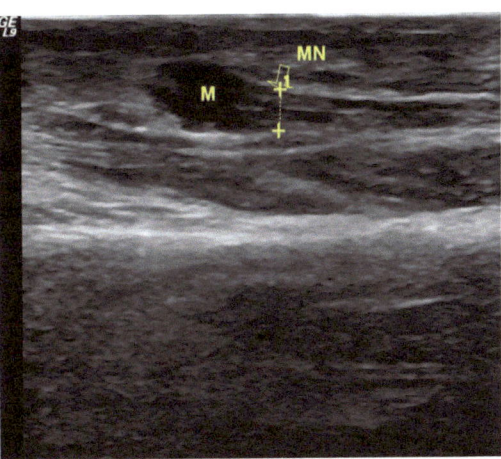

Fig. 3.8 Ultrasonogram of a fractured median nerve caused by a knife. Note: *MN* median nerve. The arrow indicates the fractured median nerve, and the Vernier calliper shows the distal part of the median nerve

Fig. 3.9 Ultrasonogram of traumatic neuroma of the median nerve. Note: *MN* median nerve; Vernier calliper shows the distal median nerve; *M* traumatic neuroma

Fig. 3.10 Ultrasonogram of carpal tunnel syndrome. Note: (**a**) R-MN is the median nerve entrapment at the right wrist; the arrow indicates the short and long axes of the thickened median nerve; (**b**) the median nerve entrapment during an operation on the wrist; the yellow arrow indicates the nerve entrapment

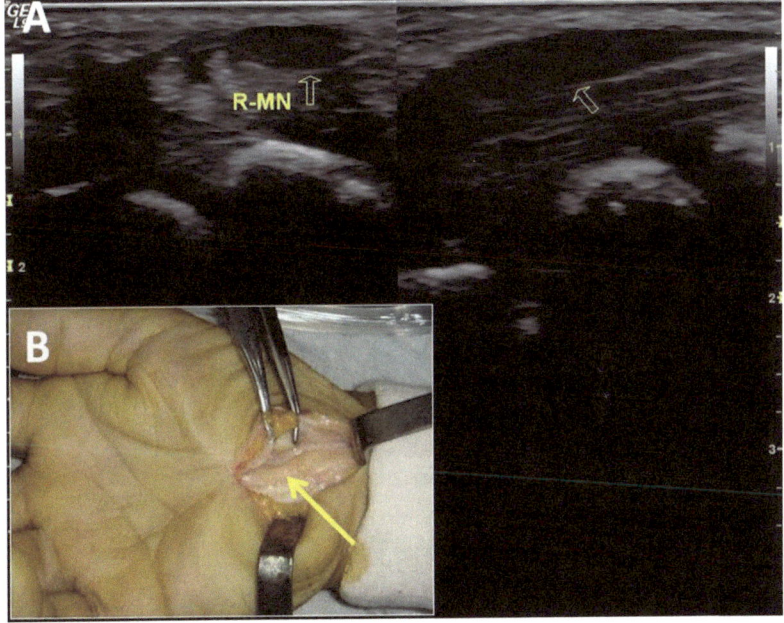

fracture causes the ulnar nerve to be pulled; medial epicondyle fracture, poor fracture reduction or osteoproliferation in the humerus may also lead to ulnar nerve injury; (2) immunological, metabolic and inflammatory lesions of the elbow joints, such as chronic rheumatoid arthritis and gouty arthritis; (3) space-occupying lesion in the cubital tunnel; (4) frequent and excessive stretching and bending of the elbow joints may cause the deltoid ligament to press against the ulnar nerve; (5) habitual ulnar nerve dislocation.

Diagnosis: (1) Cubital tunnel syndrome is common in middle-aged males, especially in manual labourers, and the common symptoms are numbness and tingling of the ring finger and the litter finger. Patients may have weak hands with the reduced gripping ability, amyotrophy, limited activities and even a malformed claw hand in the later phase. (2) The ulnar ring finger and little finger have sensory disturbances, tingling or allergy. (3) The electromyogram shows the denervation potential of the supportive muscle of the ulnar nerve, and the reduction in elbow movements and sensory nerve conduction velocity are the most valuable diagnostic findings. (4) The X-ray image shows the malunion of an old fracture at the elbows and osteoarthritis at the elbow joints.

The ultrasonogram shows that the ulnar nerve narrows at the entrapment and then enlarges at its distal and proximal ends, along with the disappearance of the neural beam echo inside and the presence of a hypoechoic structure and blurred edges; part of the lesioned nerve forms a neuroma, and the Doppler blood flow signals are increased internally (see Figs. 3.11, 3.12, and 3.13) (Video 3.4).

ER 3.4 Dynamic image and explanation of cubital tunnel syndrome and nerve cyst formation

Guyon canal syndrome, also known as Guyon syndrome, occurs when the ulnar nerve is easily compressed when it enters through the bone fibre tube or the Guyon tube at the wrists; thus, ulnar tunnel syndrome (Guyon canal syndrome) may result.

Diagnosis: (1) The ring finger and little finger will be numb and painful, with weakness and atrophy in the intrinsic muscles of the hands; even claw-like fingers may be present during the late phase. Therefore, when the patient feels impaired sensation of the ulnar ring finger, palmar little finger and ulnar palm, but has normal sensation in the dorsal metacarpal, *Guyon canal syndrome* should be considered. (2) The electromyogram shows that the lumbrical, interosseus and adductor pollicis, which are controlled by the ulnar nerve, have denervation potential, and symptoms such as restriction of wrist movements and a reduction in sensory nerve conduction velocity are helpful for a definitive diagnosis and location of this disease. (3) Ultrasonic and MRI examinations are conducive to confirming ulnar nerve morphology and the existence of a tumour in the ulnar tunnel.

Fig. 3.11 Ultrasonogram of cubital tunnel syndrome. Note: (**a**) N: long axis of the ulnar nerve. The white arrow indicates the nerve entrapment; (**b**) ulnar nerve entrapment operation. The yellow arrow indicates the entrapment

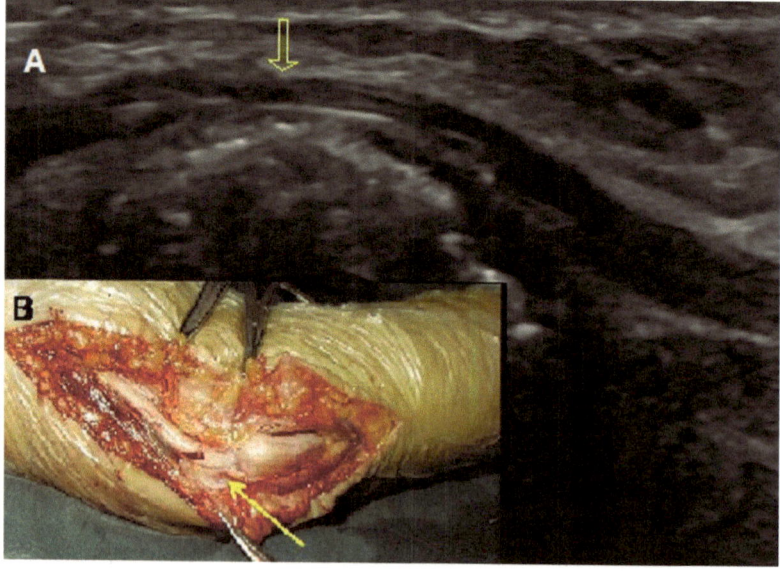

Fig. 3.12 Ultrasonogram of cubital tunnel syndrome and neural cyst. Note: the yellow arrow indicates the thickened ulnar nerve, and the Vernier calliper indicates the nerve entrapment due to the formation of a cyst

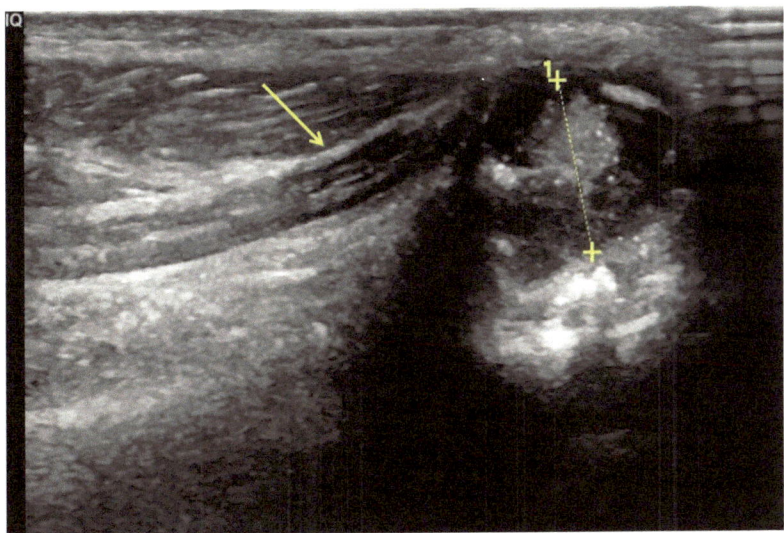

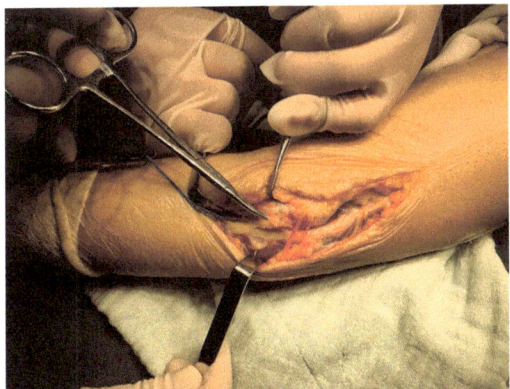

Fig. 3.13 Operation for cubital tunnel syndrome and a neural cyst

3.2.1.4 Radial Nerve Injury

The radial nerve in the upper arms is enveloped by hyperplastic fibres at the start of the lateral head of the triceps as it exits the radial groove of the humerus. Exhaustion, improper force or improper body position (for example, during a drunken sleep, the upper limb is bent and placed under the body) can cause radial nerve entrapment in the upper arms. Traumatic or iatrogenic causes also lead to radial nerve traction or fracture, thus causing injuries to different extents.

Patients often have numb hands and painful shoulders, which often expands to the dorsal part of the thumbs. During examination, the most obvious pressing pain occurs in the radial nerve in the upper arms. The electromyogram shows no abnormities in the early phase, but ultrasound can show that both ends of the affected side of the radial nerve are thicker than those of the uninjured side, while the middle part is obviously thin due to entrapment. Few cases have entrapment traces on the radial nerve [6, 7].

Diagnosis: (1) Pain in the upper arms for unobvious reasons. Patients often suffer pain below the rear of the lateral shoulder, i.e. below the rear edge of the deltoid, or in the neck and shoulders. (2) A hard stripe-like radial nerve is often palpated near the endpoint at the rear edge of the deltoid, along with obvious pressing pains stretching to the dorsum of the hand. (3) The symptoms in the late phase include muscular paralysis, difficulty in stretching the wrists and fingers, and sensory abnormities often at the dorsum of the hand and the dorsal part of the thumbs. (4) An electromyogram examination can demonstrate radial nerve injury in the upper arms, but a negative finding cannot exclude this disease.

From an ultrasonic examination, it is observed that the radial nerve at the radial groove is obviously thickened and that the radial nerve suddenly becomes thin in the radial groove when it runs into the middle half to the lower 1/3 of the upper arm (Figs. 3.14, 3.15 and 3.16).

3.2.1.5 Sciatic Nerve Injury

Piriformis syndrome refers to a kind of nerve entrapment syndrome with clinical symptoms such as numbness, pain and weak lower limbs, which are caused by stimulation and compression of the sciatic nerve due to the hyperemia, inflammation, oedema and thickening of the piriformis.

Diagnosis: (1) The middle portion of the hip may experience pain radiating to the lateral and posterior hip as well as to the lateral part of the crus. (2) The spastic piriformis can sometimes be palpated, along with obvious pressing pain that radiates to the lower limbs. (3) In cases of resistance extorsion of the hip joint, the hip pains deteriorate, while triggering numbness and pain of the lower limb on the same side (piri-

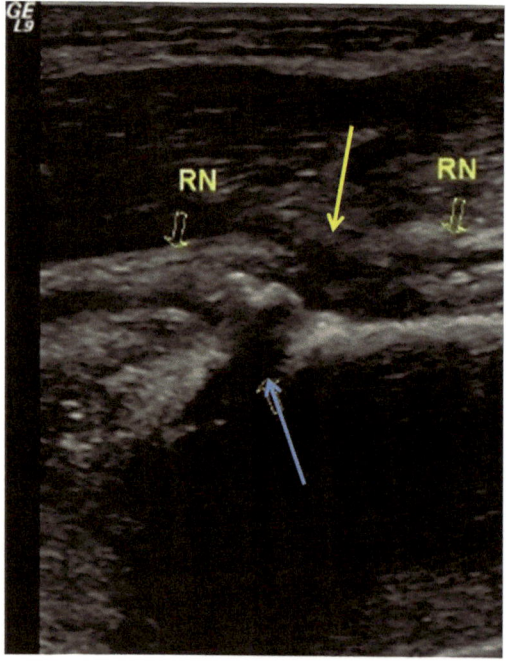

Fig. 3.14 Ultrasonogram of a radial nerve fracture in the upper arm. Note: *RN* radial nerve (yellow arrow); the blue arrow indicates fracture of the humerus, and the white arrow indicates fracture of the radial nerve

formis test). (4) An early electromyogram may not reveal abnormities, but any abnormity shown in the electromyogram is helpful for diagnosis and the definitive judgement of the nerve injury plane.

The ultrasonogram shows that the cross-sectional area of the piriformis is increased, has an abnormal shape, a hypoechoic interior, and a narrow outlet; in addition, an enlarged sciatic nerve root with oedema due to entrapment is seen, but it runs continuously (see Figs. 3.17 and 3.18). Some patients have abnormal sciatic nerves or the sciatic nerves are not clearly shown in the ultrasonogram [8, 9].

3.2.1.6 Common Peroneal Nerve Injury

The common peroneal nerve runs behind the lateral popliteal space groove, downwards to the fibular tunnel at the posterior lateral fibular head. When the volume in the fibular tunnel is decreased or the internal pressure is increased, the common peroneal nerve will experience a series of paralysis symptoms, which comprise fibular tunnel syndrome. Ultrasonic examination shows the continuity of the common peroneal nerve and changes in abnormal echoes (Figs. 3.19, 3.20 and 3.21).

3.2.1.7 Tibial Nerve Injury

Tarsal tunnel syndrome, also known as posterior tarsal tunnel syndrome, occurs as a result of tibial nerve compression as it passes through the fibrous bone sheath canals under the ligament controlled by the medial malleolus flexor. This syndrome can be divided into proximal tarsal tunnel syndrome and distal tarsal tunnel syndrome. The former means the entrapment of the main trunk of the tibial nerve, which occurs at the proximal tarsal tunnel, while the latter means entrapment of one or more branches of the tibial nerve, which often occurs at the distal tarsal tunnel, especially at the fibrous opening of the proximal abductor. The causes of entrapment include trauma, fracture of the medial malleolus, blood stasis in the posterior tibial blood vessel (especially a vein), tenosynovitis, cyst, flatfoot, blood vessel variation in muscle tendons and rheumatoid diseases. In addition, the arches of the medial feet contain

Fig. 3.15 Ultrasonogram of radial nerve constriction. Note: *RN* radial nerve. The arrow indicates constriction of the radial nerve

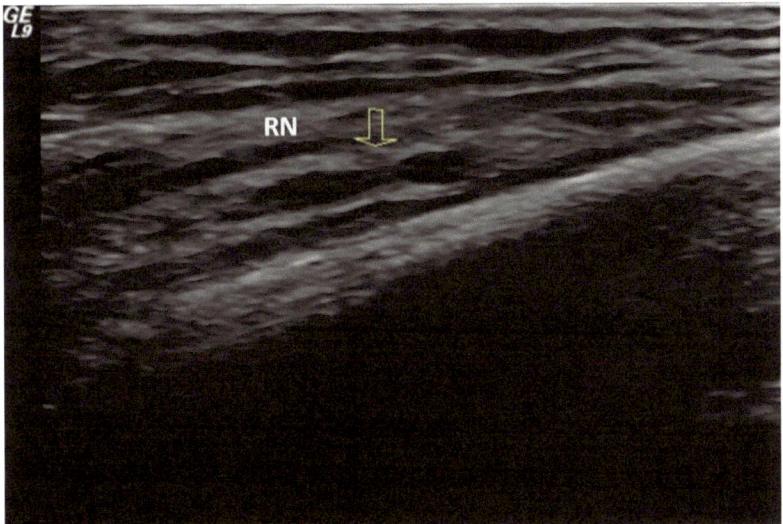

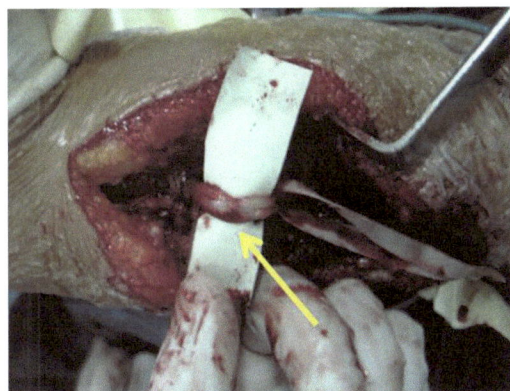

Fig. 3.16 Operation for radial nerve constriction. Note: the yellow arrow is pointing to constriction of the radial nerve during surgery

fascia to fix nerves whose lesions will cause the entrapment of the medial plantar nerve near the lower part of the navicular, which is commonly seen in jogger's feet.

3.2.2 Neurological Space-Occupying Lesions

3.2.2.1 Neurofibroma

Neurofibroma, along with other systemic diseases, is classed as neurofibromatosis, which is a type of benign peripheral nerve disease and a type of autosomal dominant genetic disease. Neurofibromatosis may be classified into two types: the common neurofibromatosis type I, known as peripheral nerve fibromatosis, involves peripheral nerves; neurofibromatosis type II involves the central nervous system.

Neurofibromatosis type I can be divided into the multiple nodular type, the plexiform type and the diffuse type based on histopathology. The multiple nodular type neurofibromatosis may occur either at larger neural trunks or at smaller cutaneous nerves, and is associated with solid masses, less bleeding and cystic degeneration. The plexiform type often occurs at the truncus and upper limbs and involves larger neural trunks and even their branches, thus forming a large number of irregular fusiform enlarged nodules of different sizes that run along the nerves. The diffuse type often occurs in the head and neck; the neural tissues grow in a diffusive manner in the skin, connective tissues and subcutaneous soft tissues, and wrap other normal tissues, while a large number of dilated blood vessels are found inside the lesions.

The manifestation of the abovementioned pathologic changes by ultrasonography: (1) Multiple nodular type: subcutaneous multiple hypoechoic nodules with clear boundaries in either a circular or ovoid shape; colour Doppler flow imaging shows few blood flow signals

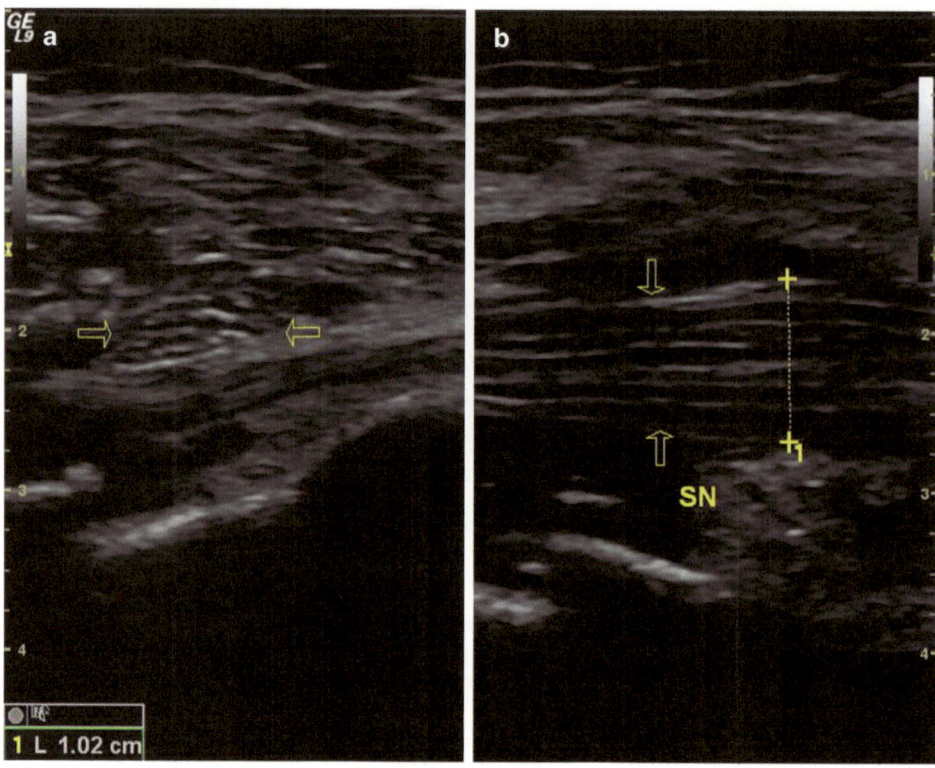

Fig. 3.17 Ultrasonogram of sciatic nerve oedema. Note: *SN* sciatic nerve; (**a**) short axis of normal sciatic nerve (arrows), (**b**) calliper and arrows indicate sciatic nerve oedema

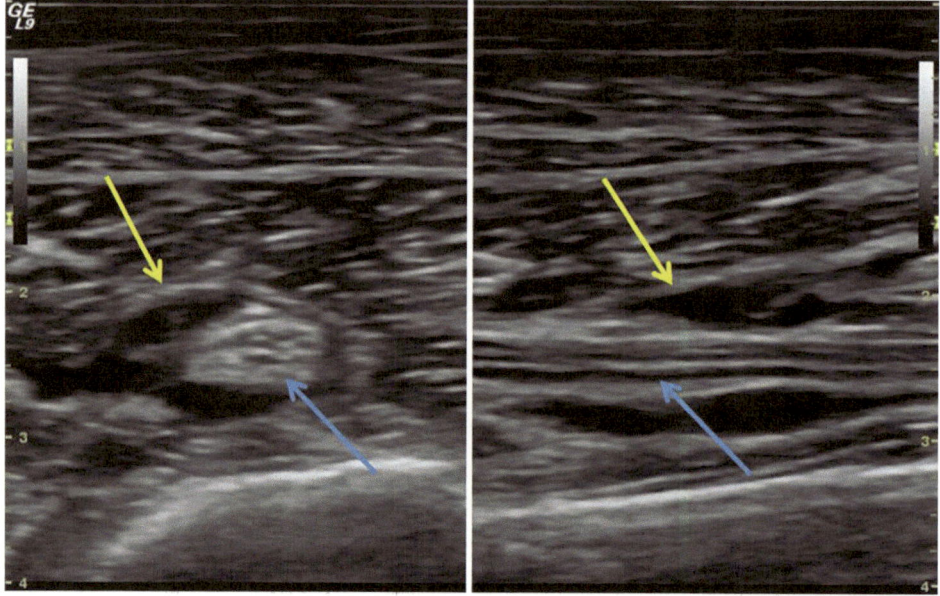

Fig. 3.18 Ultrasonogram of peripheral hydrops of the sciatic nerve. Note: the blue arrow is pointing to the short axis (left) and long axis (right) of sciatic nerve oedema, and the yellow arrow is pointing to the peripheral hydrops of the sciatic nerve

Fig. 3.19 Ultrasonogram of the long axis of common peroneal nerve injury. Note: *PN* common peroneal nerve. The arrow indicates an enlarged common peroneal nerve

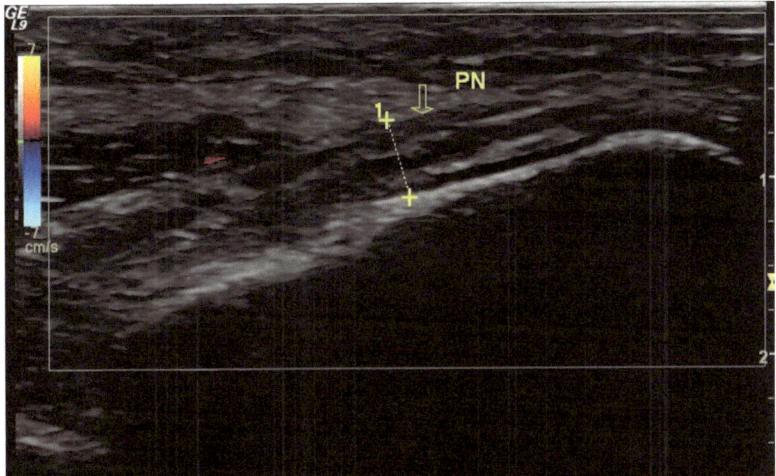

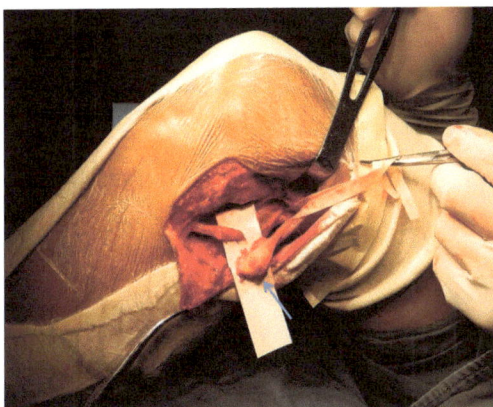

Fig. 3.20 Operation for a common peroneal nerve fracture and proximal end traumatic neuroma formation. Note: the arrow indicates the formation of a traumatic neuroma

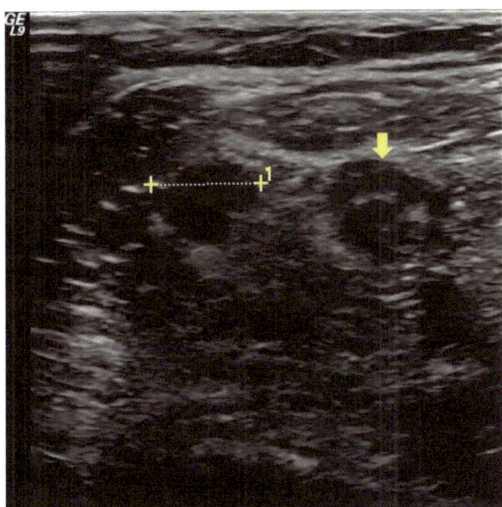

Fig. 3.21 Ultrasonogram of the short axis of common peroneal nerve injury. Note: the calliper indicates an enlarged common peroneal nerve, and the yellow arrow indicates an enlarged tibial nerve

inside the nodules. (2) The plexiform type generally involves a wide range of neural trunks, and its ultrasonogram shows that swollen, hyperplastic neural fibres, which are twisted and deformed, have bead-arrayed hypoechoic nodules connected by neural trunks in the middle; colour Doppler flow imaging shows many blood flow signals inside the nodules. (3) The diffuse type presents obviously thickened skin and a subcutaneous fat layer in the lesion area, hyperechoic change in a diffusive manner and a typical ultrasonogram of irregular scale array among hyper- and hypoechoic changes, termed a "feather-like

array"; colour Doppler imaging shows markedly increased blood flow signals in the lesion area, accompanied by aneurysm-like dilation of the vessels.

3.2.2.2 Neurilemmoma

Neurilemmoma, also known as schwannoma, is a type of benign tumour derived from Schwann cells and is also one of the most common tumours of peripheral nerves. These tumours can occur at the neural trunks or roots in any part of the body in the form of single or multiple tumours. These tumours have encapsulated membranes, and they often compress adjacent tissues and thus cause adhesion to surrounding tissue; sometimes, the tumour is accompanied by bleeding or cystic degeneration. Clinically, neurilemmoma often occurs at the neural main trunks of the head, neck and limbs, as well as the flexor sides of the arms and legs, especially the joints adjacent to the elbows, wrists and knees. Neurilemmoma grows slowly, and its clinical manifestation is painless soft tissue masses that lead to corresponding symptoms and physical signs when they compress the nerves.

The ultrasound usually shows an oval mass with a clear and smooth boundary, a hypoechoic internal structure (some have cystic degeneration), and an enhanced echo behind the mass; colour Doppler flow imaging (CDFI) shows blood flow signals inside the tumour (Figs. 3.22, 3.23, 3.24 and 3.25). The ultrasound findings mentioned

Fig. 3.22 Ultrasonogram of a neurilemmoma of the median nerve in the upper arm. Note: *MN* median nerve, and M indicates neurilemmoma

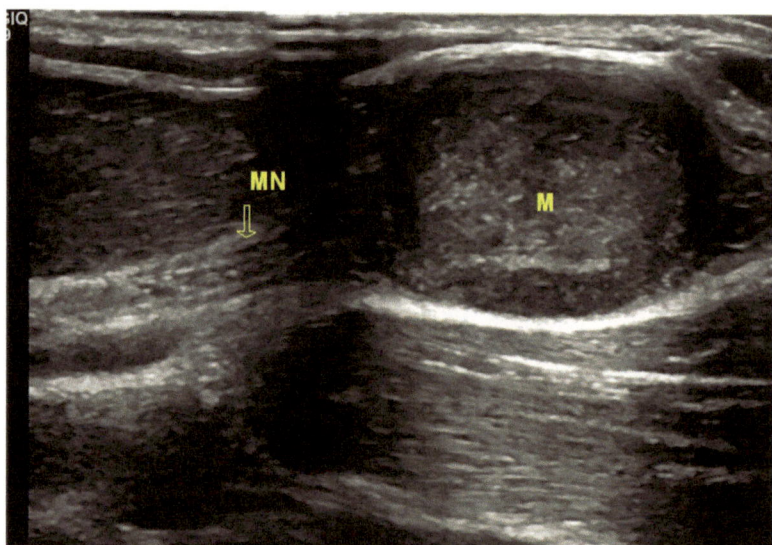

Fig. 3.23 Operation for neurilemmoma of the median nerve in the upper arm. Note: (**a**) the blue arrow is pointing to a neurilemmoma of the median nerve; (**b**) neurilemmoma after excision

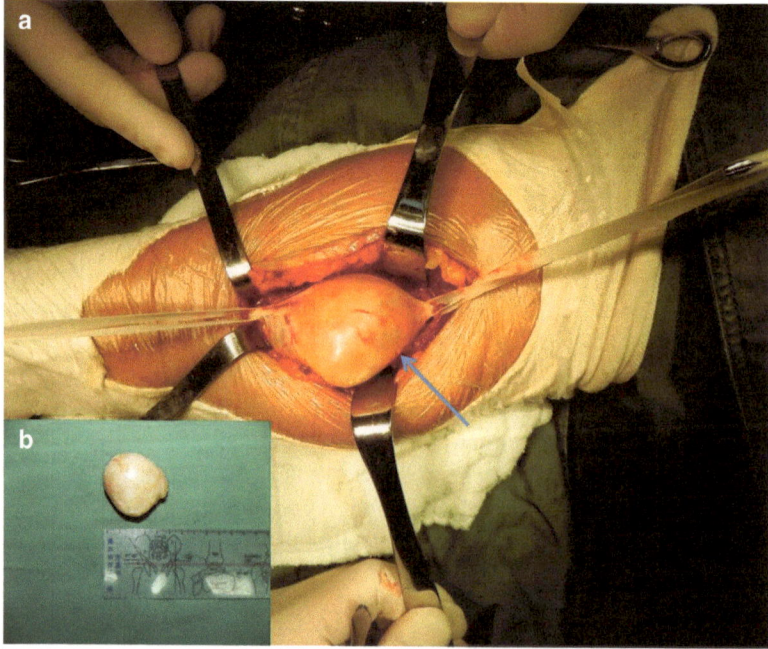

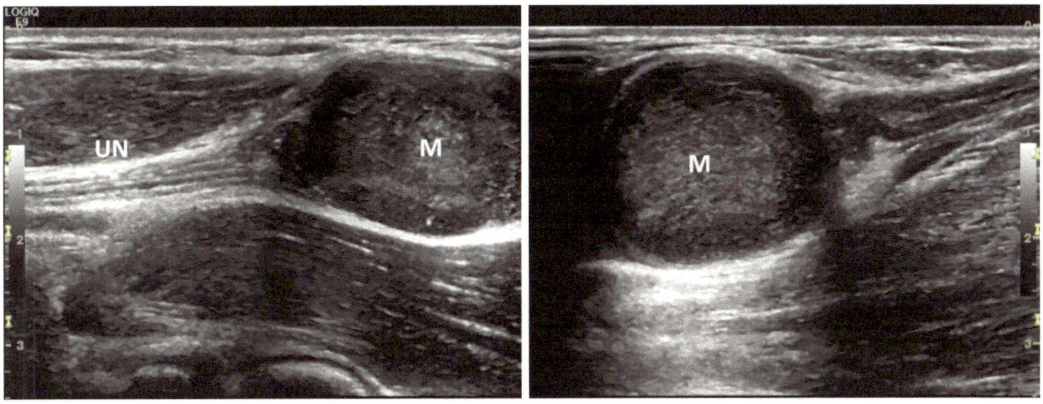

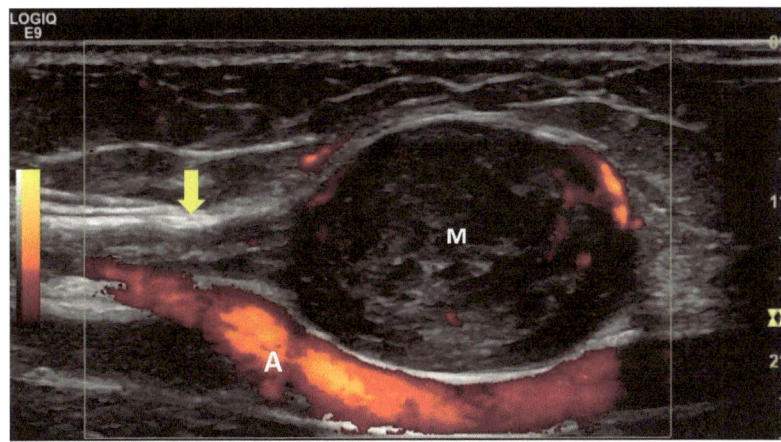

Fig. 3.24 Ultrasonogram of a neurilemmoma of the ulnar nerve in the upper arm. Note: *UN* ulnar nerve, and M indicates neurilemmoma

Fig. 3.25 Colour Doppler ultrasonogram of a neurilemmoma of the tibial nerve. Note: the yellow arrow indicates the tibial nerve, M: neurilemmoma, A: popliteal artery

above are not typical for nerve tumours, and only when the mass is observed to connect with nerves at one or both ends can it be identified as nerve tumour as opposed to other soft tissues masses. Therefore, ultrasonic examination demonstrates that the hypoechoic mass is obviously wrapped by a membrane, and if the mass runs along nerves, it might be considered a neurogenic tumour, after the exclusion of other kinds of soft tissue masses. To confirm the diagnosis, both ends of the mass should be carefully scanned to look for the connection of the neural trunk and the mass to determine the relationship between the mass and the nerve or the blood vessel. However, if the nerve is relatively small and thin, such as small nerves in the skin or subcutaneous superficial fascia, ultrasound may not be useful.

Neurilemmoma and solitary neurofibroma have a similar ultrasonogram profile, and it was previously reported that neurofibroma demonstrated more of a symmetrical growth, but in fact, masses with eccentric growth are not uncommon. Therefore, the ultrasonogram shows no obvious specificity. From two-dimensional or colour Doppler flow images, it is difficult to differentiate solitary neurofibroma and neurilemmoma, but the former rarely exhibits cystic degeneration.

3.2.2.3 Traumatic Neuroma

1. Neuroma of an interrupted nerve: the continuity of a stripe-like strong echo in the epineurium and a linear strong echo in the nerve tract is completely interrupted, and in the injured

zone a disordered hypoechoic structure is seen. The nerve at proximal end is inhomogeneous enlarged, with the normal nerves structure disappeared.

2. Stump neuroma: the neural end is enlarged in one area and presents as a hypoechoic fusiform structure.

3. Incomplete traumatic neuroma: the continuity of the nerve tract is partly broken, and the neuroma inside has an inhomogeneous hypoechoic structure; the proximal end of the neuroma partly bulges and exhibits adhesion to the surrounding soft tissues (Figs. 3.25, 3.26, 3.27, 3.28 and 3.29).

3.2.2.4 Neurolipomatosis

Neurolipomatosis, also known as neural fibrolipomatosis, is a type of rare, benign peripheral nerve lesion, which often grows in the median nerve and is accompanied by acromegaly of the affected limbs; the ultrasonogram shows hypoechoic nerve fibres and hyperechoic fatty tissues that intertwine with each other, and an enlarged nerve tract.

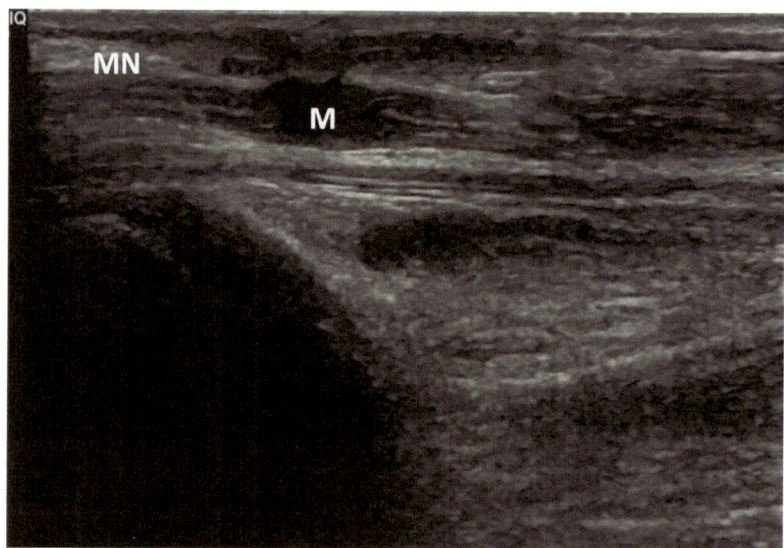

Fig. 3.26 Ultrasonogram of a traumatic neuroma of the median nerve. Note: *MN* median nerve; M: traumatic neuroma

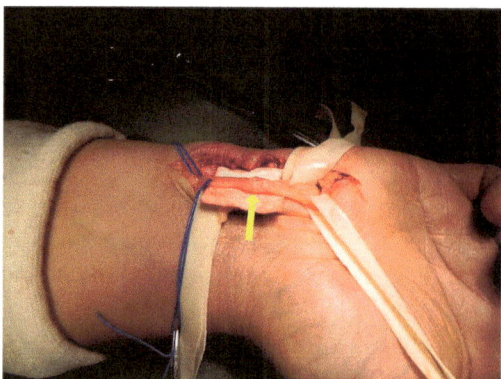

Fig. 3.27 Operation for traumatic neuroma of the median nerve. Note: the yellow arrow is pointing to the traumatic neuroma

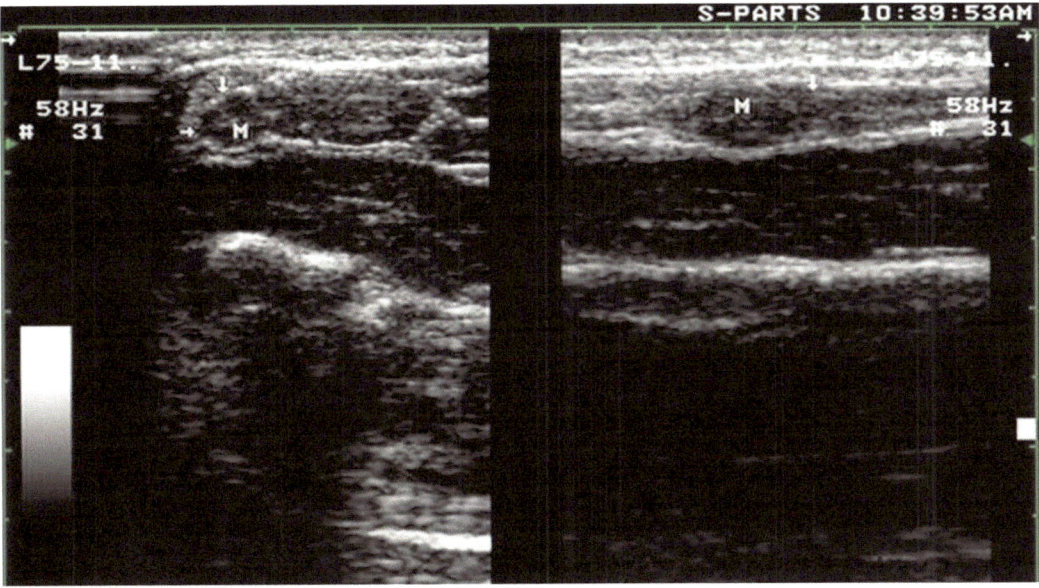

Fig. 3.28 Ultrasonogram of a traumatic neuroma of the ulnar nerve in the wrist. Note: the arrow is pointing to the short axis (left) and long axis (right) of the ulnar nerve at the wrist; M: traumatic neuroma

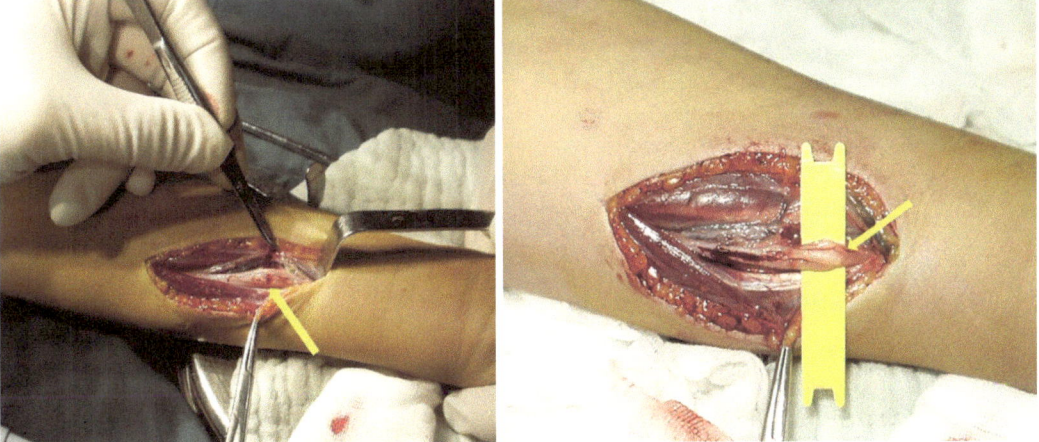

Fig. 3.29 Operation for traumatic neuroma of the ulnar nerve in the wrist. Note: the yellow arrow is pointing to the traumatic neuroma

References

1. Daga G, Kerkar PB. Brachial plexus injury after right hepatectomy. Indian J Surg Oncol. 2017;8(2):191–4.
2. Kosutic D, Gajanan K. Rare case of a liposarcoma in the brachial plexus. Ann R Coll Surg Engl. 2016;98(7):e106–8.
3. Chen AM, Yoshizaki T, Velez MA, et al. Tolerance of the brachial plexus to high-dose reirradiation. Int J Radiat Oncol Biol Phys. 2017;98(1):83–90.
4. Zheng M, Zhu Y, Zhou X, et al. Diagnosis of closed injury and neoplasm of the brachial plexus by ultrasonography. J Clin Ultrasound. 2014;42(7): 417–22.

5. Billakota S, Ruch DS, Hobson-Webb LD. Ultrasound imaging of median nerve conduit in a patient with persistent median nerve symptoms. J Clin Neurophysiol. 2018;35(1):e1–2.

6. Ljungquist KL, Martineau P, Allan C. Radial nerve injuries. J Hand Surg Am. 2015;40(1):166–72.

7. Jayendrapalan J, Ramesh VG, Karthikeyan KV, et al. Primary lymphoma of the radial nerve presenting as nerve sheath tumor. Neurol India. 2018;66(1):258–60.

8. Bracewell A, et al. Sciatic neuropathy due to popliteal space nerve block. Muscle Nerve. 2017;56(4):822–4.

9. Arányi Z, Polyák I, Tóth N, et al. Ultrasonography of sciatic nerve endometriosis. Muscle Nerve. 2016;54(3):500–5.

Dingzhang Chen, Rui Zhao, Minjuan Zheng, and Jing Wang

Informed consents were obtained from all the patients involved in cases of this chapter. Patients who under 18 years provided informed consents by their guardians.

4.1 Typical Cases of Brachial Plexus

Brachial plexus injury, a common trauma with a high rate of disability, is one of the most serious peripheral nerve injuries and generally requires surgical treatment. The accurate localization of the injured nerve by medical imaging before surgery guarantees successful treatment. Generally, traumatic brachial plexus injuries can be divided into closed injuries and open injuries. Closed injuries are often caused by stretch or crush

injury to the neck as a result of auto accidents and sport injuries (such as skiing), while open injuries are mainly caused by auto accidents and incised wounds and are usually accompanied by bone, muscle or blood vessel injuries (such as clavicle fracture, cervical spine fracture, rotator cuff tear, rupture of subclavian artery, among others). These injuries lead to avulsion, tears and injuries to the brachial plexus resulting in functional impairment of the upper arms.

Closed injuries of the brachial plexus are divided into supraclavicular injuries and subclavian injuries, and the former includes preganglionic and postganglionic injuries. Preganglionic injury, also known as brachial plexus root avulsion, refers to the filiform structural rupture of the spinal nerve as a constituent of the brachial plexus at the spinal cord, which causes neuronal damage or death. This root avulsion is the most serious brachial plexus injury, as it can cause permanent disability to patients' limbs. Postganglionic injuries include injuries in roots, trunks (superior, medial and inferior trunk), cords (medial, lateral and posterior cord) and at the origins of the main nerves in the upper limbs. As the slightest injury, brachial plexus usually maintains its structural integrity in cases of postganglionic injury, with a complete neuromechanism and temporary absence of functions. These injuries may cause the failure or temporary loss of nerve conduction function due to stretched and tightened nerve fibre bundles, with axonal degeneration, epineurium

Supplementary Information The online version contains supplementary material available at https://doi.org/10.1007/978-981-15-2704-3_4.

D. Chen (✉) · M. Zheng · J. Wang
Department of Ultrasound, Xijing Hospital, Fourth Military Medical University, Xi'an, Shaanxi, China

R. Zhao
Hand Surgery, Xijing Hospital, Fourth Military Medical University, Xi'an, China

oedema, peripheral bleeding and adhesion, even organization, and fibrous scar formation [1].

Since it is difficult for neurons to regenerate, the treatment effects of brachial plexus injury are not very satisfactory due to the higher injury position and partial permanent neuronal degeneration. The diagnosis and treatment of brachial plexus injury is still a difficult clinical problem. Thus, early diagnosis is crucial for the prognosis and curative effect of treatment.

4.1.1   Preganglionic Injury (Cases 1–5)

Preganglionic injury of the brachial plexus, which cannot recover by itself, refers to the rupture at the filiform structures of the anterior and posterior roots of the cervical nerve in the vertebral canal. Its pathological basis is that the cerebrospinal fluid flows along the nerve root to the epidural or outer vertebral canal in cases of nerve root avulsion or nerve sheath rupture. However, injuries of the surrounding soft tissues or the formation of scars may restrict flow or warp the cerebrospinal fluid, and thus pseudocysts are formed at the affected side of the intervertebral foramen; they may even extend to the axilla in severe cases. Such findings can be regarded as the basis of its imaging diagnosis.

Preganglionic injuries are more severe in terms of damage and are often accompanied by coma, multiple fractures of the neck, shoulders and upper limbs, and continuous severe pain. The main points for ultrasonic diagnosis are as follows: the nerve from the origin of the brachial plexus root narrows and then disappears or it is swollen and oedematous at its distal end, with its continuity destroyed. Simultaneously, a cystic mass grows beside the vertebral canal due to cystic accumulation of cerebrospinal fluid inside or beside the neural canal.

Case 1

A male patient, aged 20 years with a history of injury, experienced a loss of movement functions and sensation disturbance on his left upper arm for more than 2 months. A specialized physical examination revealed the following: an immobile, hard mass 4 cm × 3 cm in his left neck could be palpated, with slight pressing pain and was accompanied by numbness and obvious muscular atrophy of his left

upper limb, and gravitational dislocation of his left shoulder joint. Electromyogram: no waves for the left median nerve, ulnar nerve, radial nerve, musculocutaneous nerve or axillary nerve, which indicated serious injuries. MRI: left brachial plexus injury accompanied by peripheral tissue contusion, spinal cord degeneration of the corresponding plane, and benign cystic degeneration at the left cervical root on the intervertebral plane between C6 and C7.

Ultrasound: the brachial plexus exited the roots of C5, C6 and C7 and narrowed to 0.2–0.3 cm in diameter and ran downwards to an echoless zone of 2.6 cm × 3.6 cm with a clear boundary 3.0 cm away from C6; the brachial plexus from C8 was not shown, and adjacent to the vertebral canal and vertebral artery at C8 was an echoless zone of approximately 2.5 cm × 0.9 cm. The ulnar nerve and radial nerve at the axilla ran continuously without obvious abnormalities. Ultrasound findings: in left brachial plexus injuries, oedema of the nerves at the superior, medial and inferior trunks was observed, and there was no nerve root from C8; a cystic mass (cyst) beside the C8 vertebral canal was also observed. Preganglionic injury was suspected (Figs. 4.1, 4.2, 4.3, 4.4 and 4.5) (Video 4.1).

Operation: C5 to T1 nerve roots on the left side are completely removed from the subclavian plane, with cerebrospinal fluid cysts forming at two places. Preganglionic injury is determined from the electromyogram during surgery.

ER 4.1 Dynamic image and explanation of the case of preganglionic root avulsion of the brachial plexus

Case 2
See (Figs. 4.6, 4.7 and 4.8) (Video 4.2).

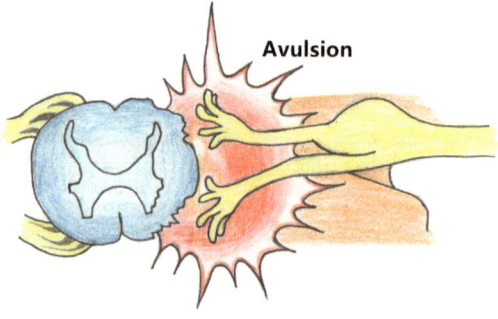

Fig. 4.1 Schematic of root avulsion of the brachial plexus

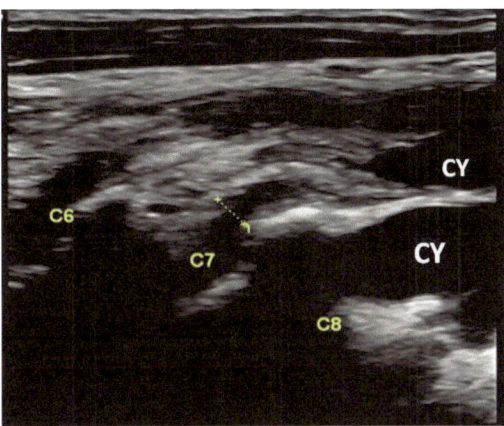

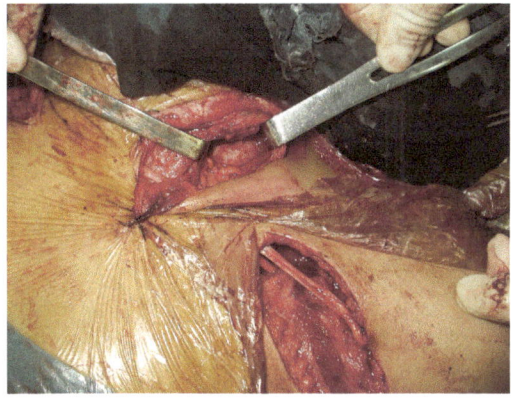

Fig. 4.5 Image of the operation on a preganglionic root avulsion of the brachial plexus

Fig. 4.2 Ultrasonogram of preganglionic root avulsion of the brachial plexus at the C8 level. Note: the nerve root from C6 and C7 becomes thin, and no nerve root exits C8; CY: formation of cerebrospinal fluid cyst

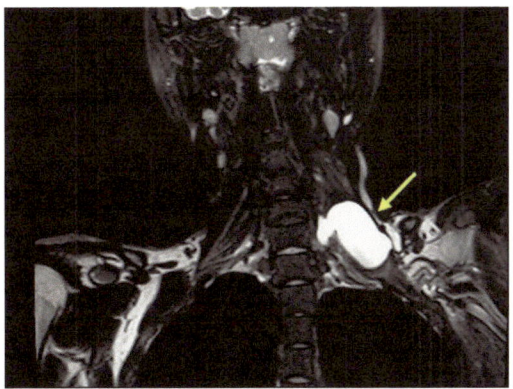

Fig. 4.3 MRI coronal image of preganglionic root avulsion of the brachial plexus. Note: the yellow arrow is pointing to the C8 cerebrospinal fluid cyst

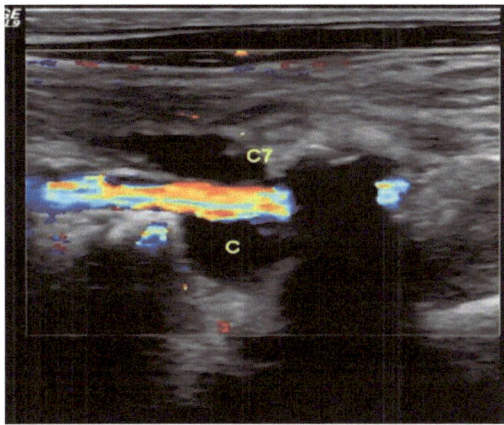

Fig. 4.6 Ultrasonogram of preganglionic root avulsion of the brachial plexus at the C7 level. Note: C indicates a cyst

ER 4.2 Dynamic image and explanation of preganglionic root avulsion of the brachial plexus

Case 3
See (Figs. 4.9, 4.10 and 4.11) (Video 4.3).

ER 4.3 Dynamic image and explanation of preganglionic root avulsion of the brachial plexus

Case 4
See (Figs. 4.12, 4.13 and 4.14).

Case 5
See (Figs. 4.15 and 4.16) (Video 4.4).

ER 4.4 Dynamic image and explanation of total brachial plexus injury

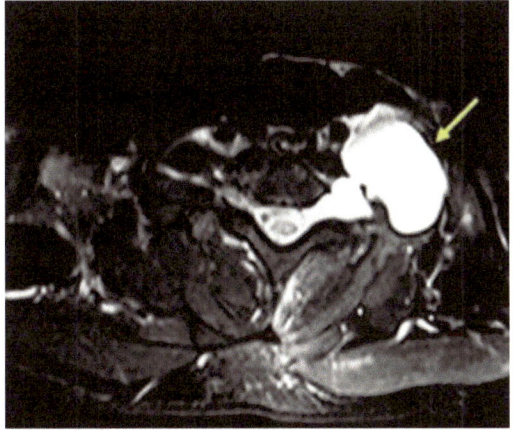

Fig. 4.4 MRI cross-sectional image of preganglionic root avulsion of the brachial plexus

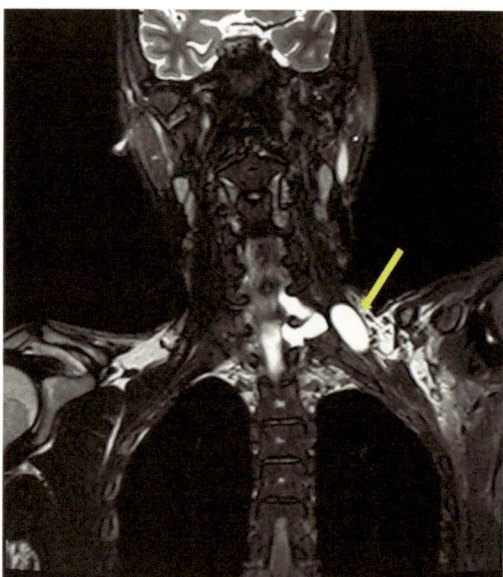

Fig. 4.7 MRI of preganglionic root avulsion of the brachial plexus. Note: the high intensity zone indicated by the yellow arrow is a cyst

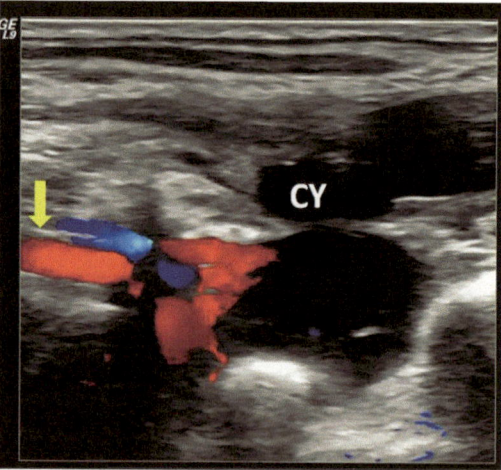

Fig. 4.9 Ultrasonogram of preganglionic root avulsion of the brachial plexus (involving the whole brachial plexus). Note: the yellow arrow is pointing to the vertebral artery, and CY is the cyst adjacent to the vertebral artery

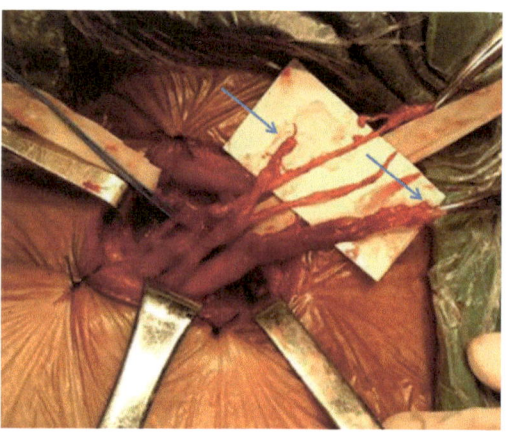

Fig. 4.8 Image of the operation on a preganglionic root avulsion of the brachial plexus. Note: the blue arrow is pointing to a root avulsion of the brachial plexus

4.1.2 Postganglionic Injury (Cases 6–12)

Postganglionic injury refers to extraforaminal root and trunk injuries of a nerve, with symptoms of different degrees of disturbance and/or amyotrophy in upper limb movement and sensation. The main points for ultrasonic exami-

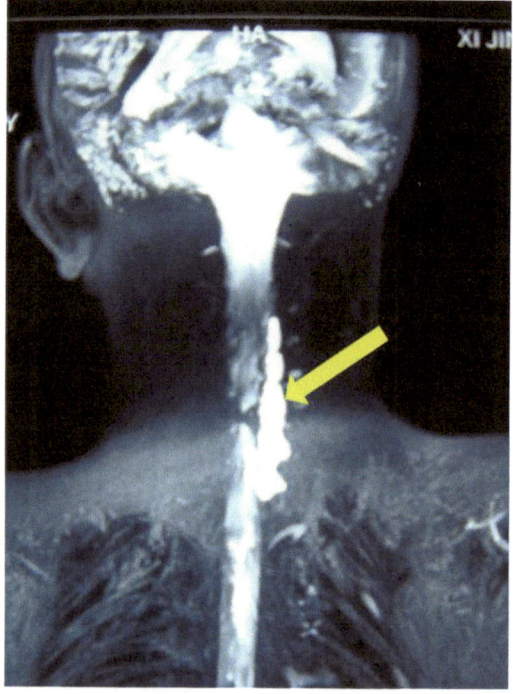

Fig. 4.10 CT angiography image of the spinal cord in a case of brachial plexus root avulsion. Note: the yellow arrow is pointing to leakage of the contrast agent

nation are as follows: the brachial plexus exits the nerve roots as usual and runs continuously with different degrees of thickening or oedema

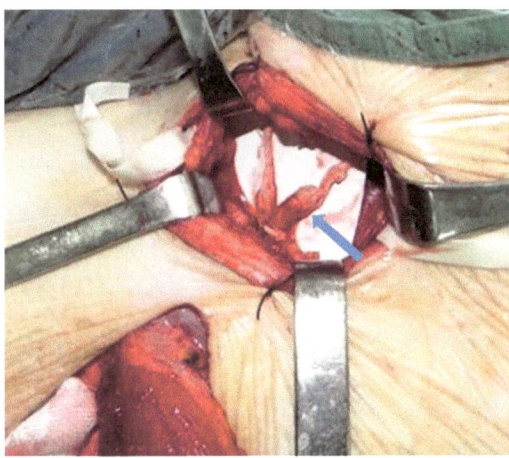

Fig. 4.11 Image of the operation for root avulsion of the brachial plexus. Note: the blue arrow is pointing to root avulsion of the brachial plexus

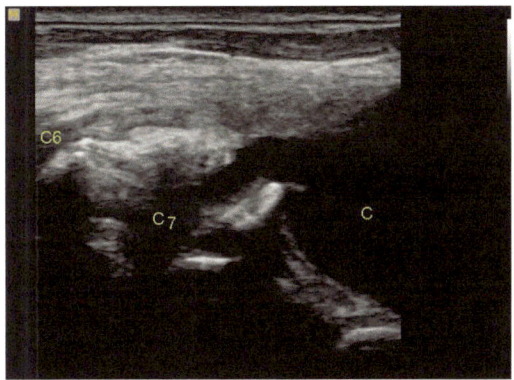

Fig. 4.12 Ultrasonogram of preganglionic root avulsion of the brachial plexus at the C5–C7 level. Note: no nerve root exits C6 and C7; C indicates a cyst

or adhesion of the brachial plexus trunk beside the subclavian artery and the nerves on the level of nerve bundles; alternatively, partial breakage of nerve continuity is seen on the subclavian artery level.

Case 6

A male patient, aged 53 years with a current medical history: the patient experienced paraesthesia and movement restriction of his right upper limb after an injury sustained 2 months prior. Now, the patient's right upper limb has lost sensation and movement functions.

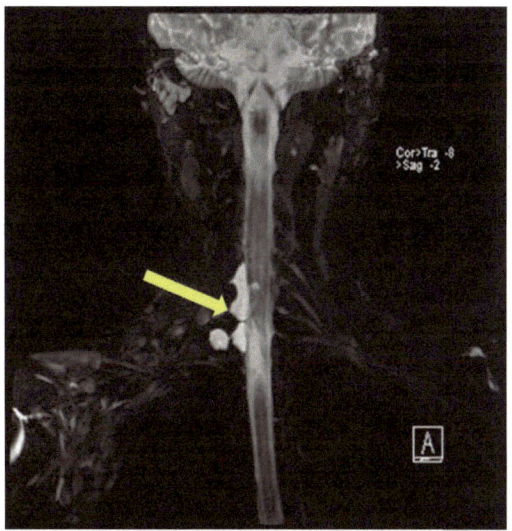

Fig. 4.13 MRI of preganglionic root avulsion of the brachial plexus. Note: the yellow arrow is pointing to cerebrospinal fluid

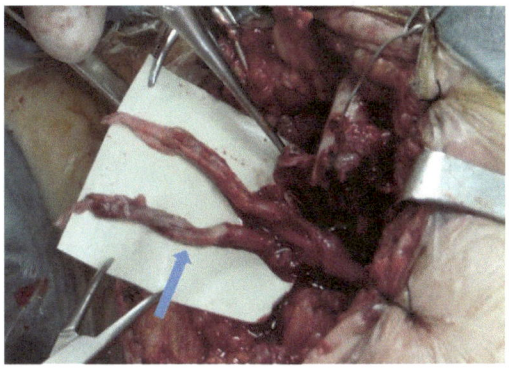

Fig. 4.14 Image of the operation for preganglionic root avulsion of the brachial plexus. Note: the blue arrow is pointing to the root avulsion

Specialized physical examination showed the following: his right shoulder was deformed, the muscle force of the right upper limb was a grade 0, the right shoulder and deltoid area had amyotrophy, and the joints of the right shoulder, elbow, wrist and right hand lost their active movement functions; the face and limb on the right side exhibited hypaesthesia, the muscle force of the right pectoralis major muscle and latissimus dorsal muscle was grade 0, and the supraspinatus, infraspinatus and del-

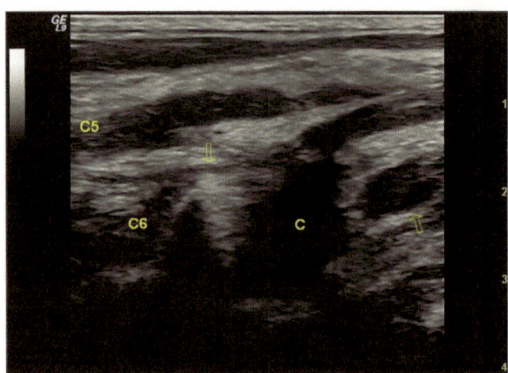

Fig. 4.15 Ultrasonogram of total brachial plexus injury (C7 cerebrospinal fluid cyst formation). Note: C indicates a cyst, and no nerve root exits C5 and C6

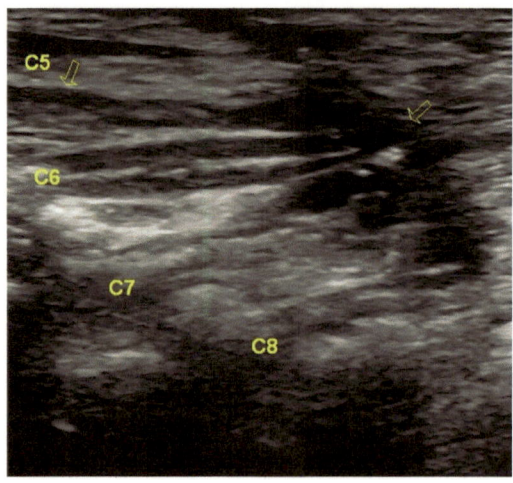

Fig. 4.17 Ultrasonogram of postganglionic rupture of the brachial plexus (total brachial plexus). Note: the brachial plexus from C5, C6, C7 and C8 are enlarged at the roots, and the arrow is pointing to the rupture of the distal end at the nerve trunk level

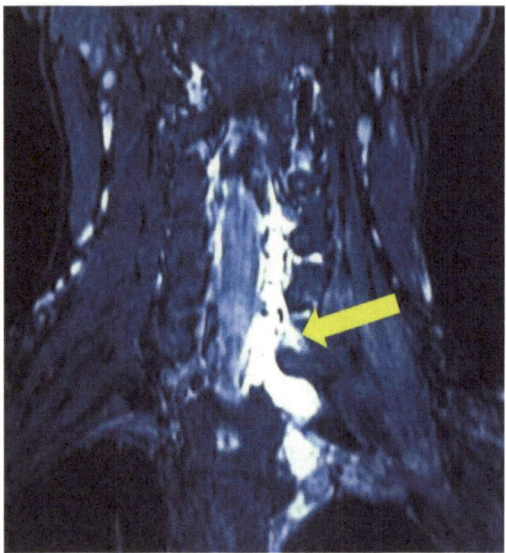

Fig. 4.16 MRI of total brachial plexus injury (C7 cerebrospinal fluid cyst formation). Note: the yellow arrow is pointing to leakage of cerebrospinal fluid

toid muscles on the right shoulder appeared to have amyotrophy and were collapsed; the tendon reflex of the biceps brachii muscle was left/right =−/+, while that of the triceps brachii muscle was left/right =−/+; at the right supraclavicular fossa and infraclavicular fossa was Tinel's sign (+), while the right side was Horner's sign (+).

Electromyogram: The electrophysiological profile of the right total brachial plexus injury likely involved preganglionic injury of the total brachial plexus.

Ultrasound: the right brachial plexus exited the C5, C6, C7 and C8 nerve roots and ran continuously and measured 0.50 cm, 0.47 cm, 0.51 cm and 0.48 cm in diameter, respectively. Rupture at the neural trunk level occurred, and the fractured ends exhibited adhesion and the beam structure disappeared. Ultrasound finding: postganglionic rupture of the right brachial plexus.

Operation: broken brachial plexus was found at the C5–C8 trunk level and was repaired after local debridement (Figs. 4.17, 4.18, 4.19 and 4.20) (Video 4.5).

ER 4.5 Dynamic image and explanation of postganglionic injury of the brachial plexus

Case 7
See (Fig. 4.21) (Video 4.6).

ER 4.6 Dynamic image and explanation of postganglionic (superior trunk) injury of the brachial plexus

Case 8
See (Figs. 4.22 and 4.23) (Video 4.7).

ER 4.7 Dynamic image and explanation of post-ganglionic (middle-superior trunk) injury of the brachial plexus

Case 9
See (Fig. 4.24) (Video 4.8).

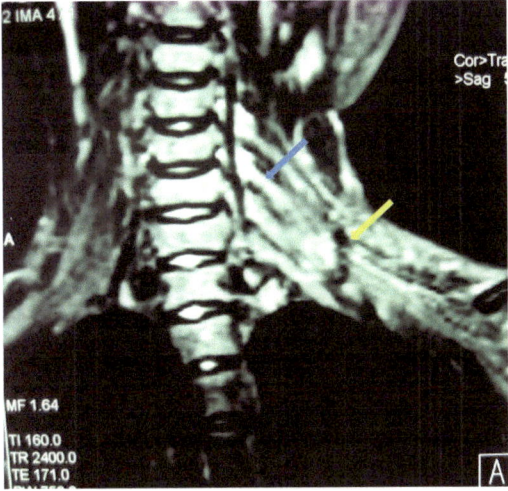

Fig. 4.18 MRI of postganglionic rupture of the brachial plexus. Note: the blue arrow is pointing to the C6 nerve root, and the yellow arrow is pointing to the rupture of the brachial plexus at the trunk level

ER 4.8 Dynamic image and explanation of post-ganglionic (middle-inferior trunk) injury of the brachial plexus

Case 10
See (Figs. 4.25, 4.26 and 4.27) (Video 4.9).

ER 4.9 Dynamic image and explanation of brachial plexus postganglionic (trunk level) injury

Case 11
See (Figs. 4.28, 4.29 and 4.30) (Video 4.10).

ER 4.10 Dynamic image and explanation of postganglionic (cord level) injury of the brachial plexus

Case 12
See (Figs. 4.31 and 4.32) (Video 4.11).

ER 4.11 Dynamic image and explanation of bundle level injury (musculocutaneous nerve) of the brachial plexus

Summary According to their anatomical positions, brachial plexus injuries include pregangli-

Fig. 4.19 Image of the operation for the postganglionic rupture of the brachial plexus (before suture). Note: the yellow arrow is pointing to the fractured end before suture

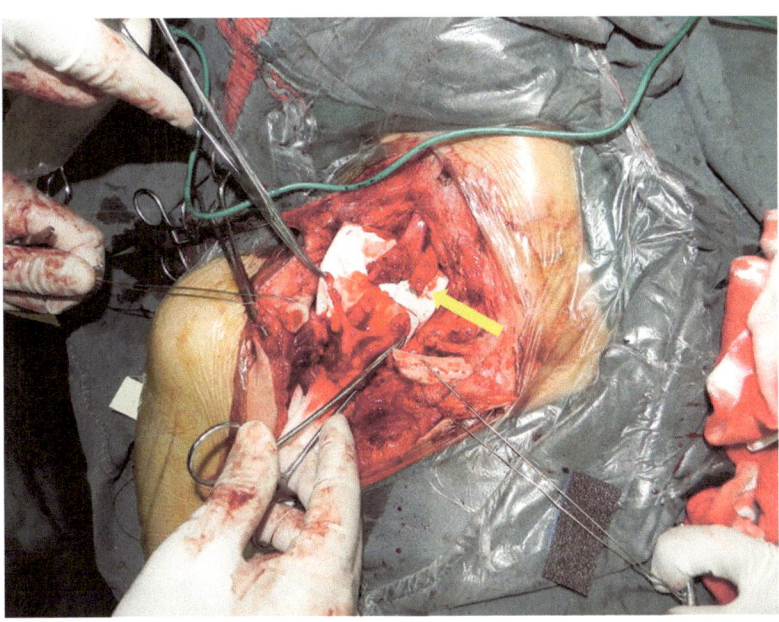

Fig. 4.20 Image of the operation for the postganglionic rupture of the brachial plexus (after suture). Note: the yellow arrow is pointing to the nerve after suture

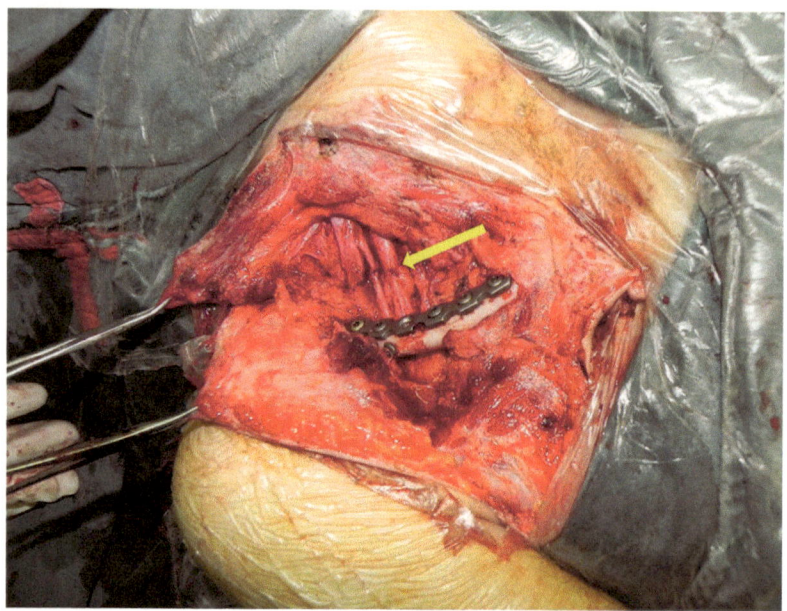

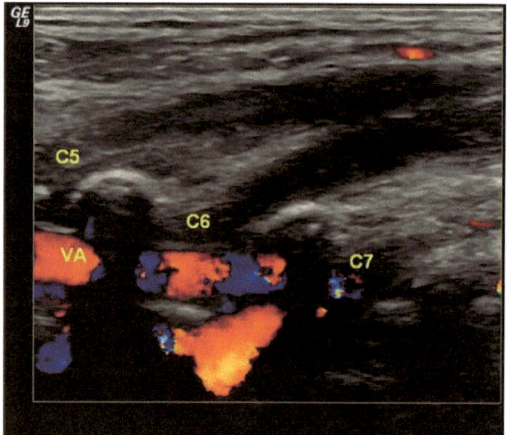

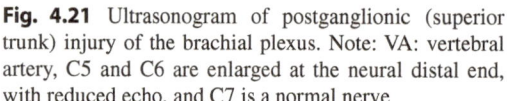

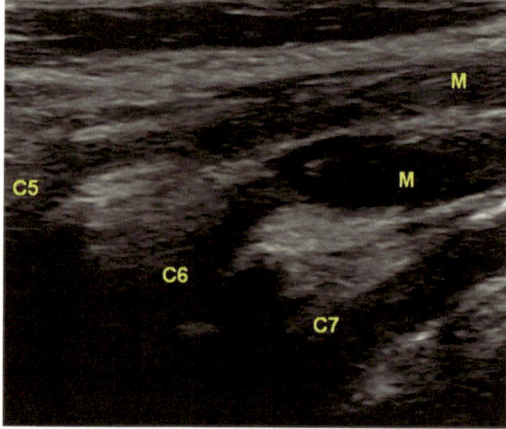

Fig. 4.21 Ultrasonogram of postganglionic (superior trunk) injury of the brachial plexus. Note: VA: vertebral artery, C5 and C6 are enlarged at the neural distal end, with reduced echo, and C7 is a normal nerve

Fig. 4.22 Ultrasonogram of postganglionic (medial-superior trunk) injury of the brachial plexus. Note: brachial plexus roots exit C5, C6 and C7, M is significantly enlarged C5 and C6 nerves, with hypoechoic change

onic injuries and postganglionic injuries by diagnosis. Different injury positions have significantly different treatment methods and prognoses. Therefore, the definite diagnosis is of great reference value for deciding the clinical treatment. High-frequency ultrasound can clearly show the different states, running paths and diameters of brachial plexus injuries. The C5-C8 nerve were shown as circle structures in the scalene muscle

space from the transverse view, which facilitates the diagnosis in that nerve roots from C5 to C8 narrow and gradually disappear due to injury or other reasons; injury signs such as neural enlargement, oedema, cystic aggregation of cerebrospinal fluid in the neural canal, meningocele, and cyst formation can also be clearly shown. As per the diagnosis, postganglionic injuries include injuries of the superior, middle and inferior trunks

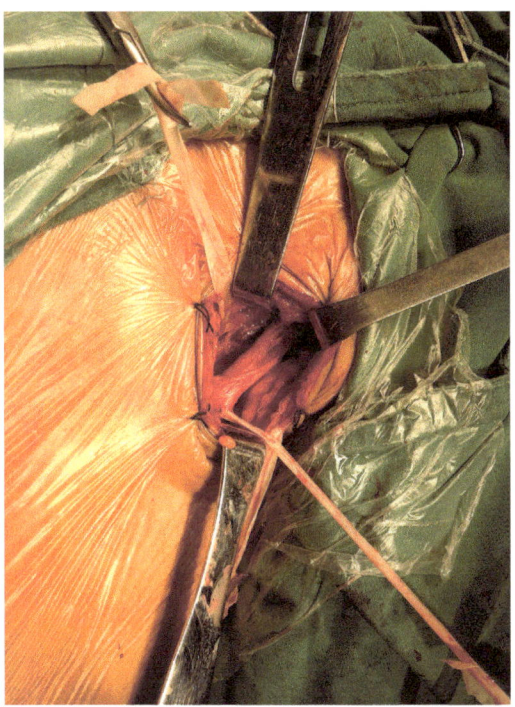

Fig. 4.23 Image of the operation for postganglionic (middle-superior trunk) injury of the brachial plexus

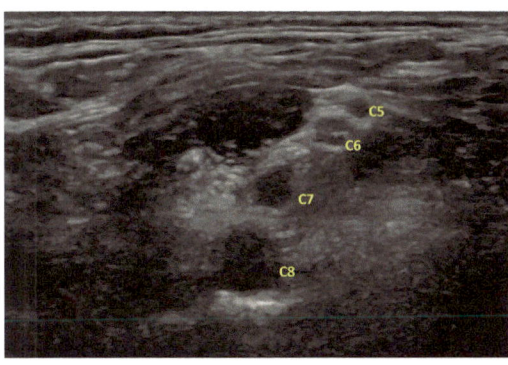

Fig. 4.24 Ultrasonogram of postganglionic (middle-inferior trunk) injury of the brachial plexus. Note: C7 and C8 nerve roots are injured, while C5 and C6 nerve roots are normal

and at the cord level. The specific and definite locations of the injuries offer important diagnostic value to clinical treatment [2].

Notes 1. The basis to judge preganglionic and postganglionic injuries is whether the nerve roots exiting the intervertebral foramen are continuous;

2. That the nerves at the roots are thin, have interrupted continuity, or disappear, with unclear display by ultrasound, in addition to the cystic aggregation of cerebrospinal fluid beside the neural canal, are features of preganglionic injury. 3. After exiting the intervertebral foramen, the nerves with complete continuity at the roots exhibit thickening, tumour-like changes, interrupted continuity, scar and adhesion at the distal end, which are the features of postganglionic injury.

4.1.3   Neurilemmoma of the Brachial Plexus (Cases 13–20)

Neurilemmoma of the brachial plexus is a type of benign tumour derived from the brachial plexus neurolemma, but malignant lesions are rarely seen. This tumour develops slowly with nontypical clinical symptoms. At the early stage, there may be no symptoms or symptoms may consist of only a painless mass at the supraclavicular, subclavian or axillary region around the neck. As the mass grows, local pain and swelling may emerge. When the tumour is palpated, the patient may feel numbness and pain radiating to the distal ends of the limbs. By physical examination, the lump is mostly a round or oval solid mass, with a hard texture, smooth surface, clear boundary, no cohesion with surrounding tissues, and certain mobility. Tinel's sign is usually positive, and occasionally, Horner's sign is positive.

The main points for ultrasonic diagnosis are as follows: 1. a typical tumour of this type has a clear boundary with a circular or ovoid hypoechoic structure and is enveloped by a hyperechoic membrane; 2. the tumour has a homogeneous echo inside and an increased echo behind; 3. the tumour is derived from the neural edge, the nerve cord runs along its profile, and colour Doppler shows blood flow signals inside; 4. rat tail sign: the tumour grows along the nerve trunk, and both ends extend and thus form a vimineous hypoechoic belt, whose shape resembles a rat tail.

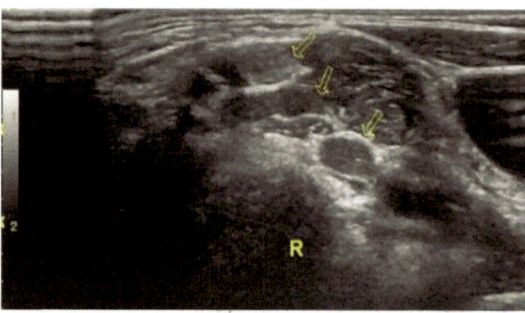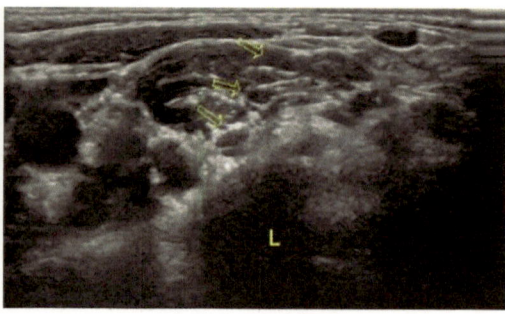

Fig. 4.25 Ultrasonogram of postganglionic (trunk level) injury of the brachial plexus. Note: R: right side, the arrow is pointing to the enlarged nerve at the trunk level of the brachial plexus; L: left (contralateral) side, the arrow is pointing to normal brachial plexus

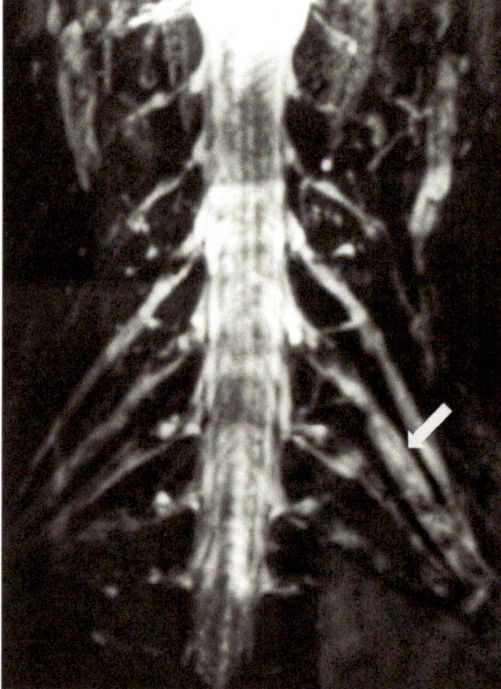

Fig. 4.26 MRI of postganglionic (trunk level) injury of the brachial plexus. Note: the yellow arrow is pointing to the affected side of an enlarged nerve with oedema

Case 13

A male patient, aged 50 years, visited the clinic for a lump in the right neck that appeared over 10 days prior. Recently, his hands were numb, especially the radial side of the right hand. Physical examination: a hard, immobile mass of 5 cm × 3 cm was found on the right side of the neck, along with pressing pain and numbness of his right upper limb. MRI examination: a cystic space-occupying lesion was observed on the right C6–C7 intervertebral plane/where the C6 nerve root runs.

Ultrasound: the right brachial plexus began and ran smoothly, the C7 intervertebral foramen was obviously enlarged and extended outwards, presenting a solid lesion of approximately 5 cm × 2.7 cm; C5, C6 and C8 nerves had no obvious abnormities. Ultrasonic diagnosis: C7 neurilemmoma in the right neck (Figs. 4.33, 4.34, 4.35 and 4.36) (Video 4.12).

Operation: a soft mass 5.0 cm × 2.2 cm × 2.2 cm wrapped in the epineurium of the upper trunk of the brachial plexus was seen on the right side of the neck. The mass was completely separated from the epineurium by decollement. The mass was diagnosed as a right cervical neurilemmoma according to postoperative pathologic analysis.

ER 4.12 Dynamic image and explanation of a C7 neurilemmoma of the brachial plexus

Case 14

See (Figs. 4.37, 4.38, 4.39 and 4.40) (Video 4.13).

ER 4.13 Dynamic image and explanation of a C5 neurilemmoma of the brachial plexus

Case 15

See (Figs. 4.41, 4.42 and 4.43).

Case 16

See (Fig. 4.44) (Videos 4.14 and 4.15).

Fig. 4.27 Image of the operation for postganglionic (trunk level) injury of the brachial plexus. Note: the yellow arrow is pointing to the enlarged nerve with oedema at the trunk level

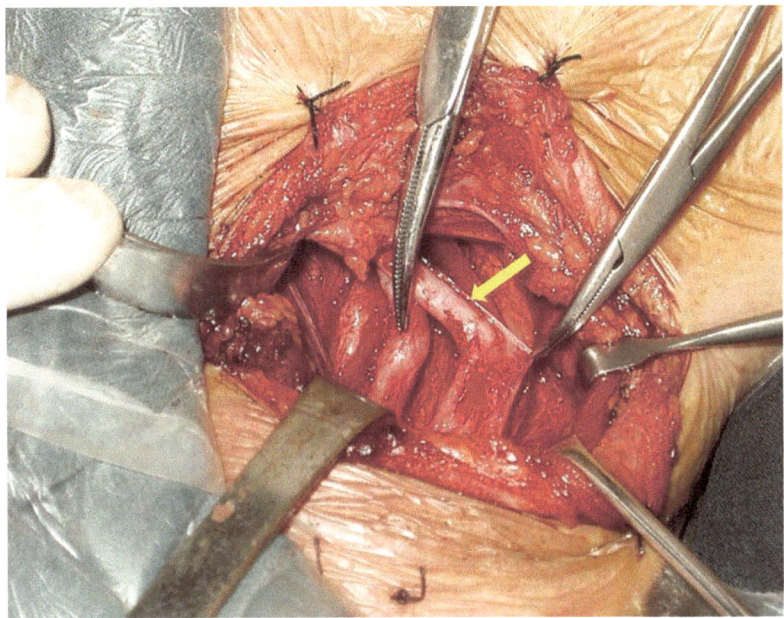

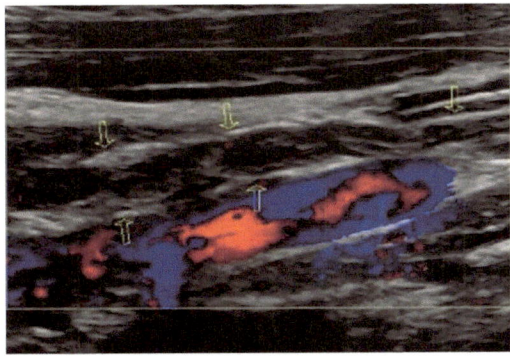

Fig. 4.28 Ultrasonogram of postganglionic cord level injury of the brachial plexus. Note: the arrow is pointing to the enlarged nerve with oedema at the cord level

ER 4.14 Dynamic image and explanation of the cystic change in a C5 schwannoma of the brachial plexus

ER 4.15 Dynamic image and explanation of contrast-enhanced ultrasound (CEUS) of cystic changes in a C5 schwannoma of the brachial plexus

Case 17
See (Figs. 4.45, 4.46 and 4.47).

Case 18
See (Figs. 4.48 and 4.49) (Videos 4.16 and 4.17).

ER 4.16 Dynamic image and explanation of a C5 schwannoma of the brachial plexus

Case 19 ER 4.17 Dynamic image and explanation of polyneuropathy in the intervertebral foramen of the brachial plexus

Case 20
See (Figs. 4.50 and 4.51) (Video 4.18).

ER 4.18 Dynamic image and explanation of a C8 neurilemmoma of the brachial plexus

Summary The brachial plexus neurilemmoma (schwannoma) at the paravertebral space mainly contains the cervical plexus and brachial plexus rather than lymphoid tissues. The complex structure seen here often leads to misdiagnosis and even the incorrect excision of the tumour and its nerve trunk, which results in further iatrogenic brachial plexus injury. Therefore, the correct diagnosis for the mass shown here is important for subsequent clinical treatment.

Notes for the diagnosis of brachial plexus schwannoma: 1. The main manifestation of brachial plexus schwannoma is the rat tail sign, which is essentially the nerve branches connected

Fig. 4.29 Ultrasonogram of a thrombus in the axillary artery. Note: L (left) is affected side, TH: thrombus, due to blood vessel damage; R (right) is a normal contralateral axillary artery

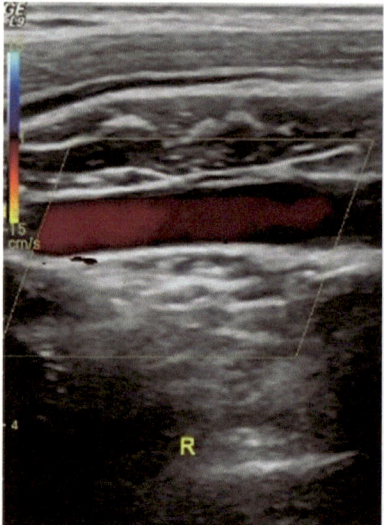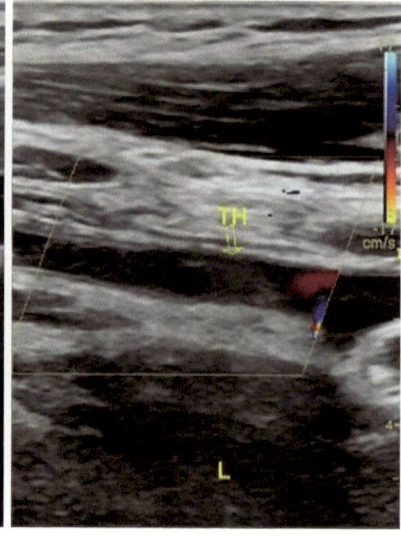

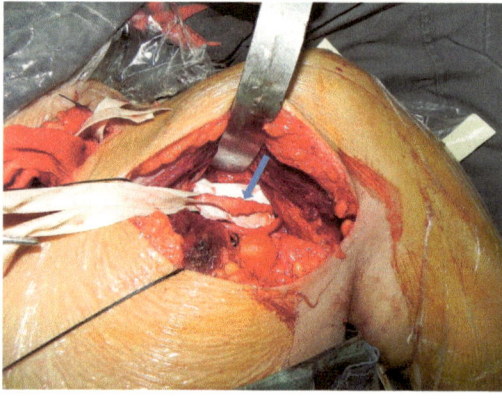

Fig. 4.30 Image of the operation for postganglionic cord level (axillary nerve) injury of the brachial plexus. Note: the blue arrow is pointing to the neural injury

to the tumour. The main ultrasonic question in patients in whom schwannoma is suspected is to judge whether the rat tail sign exists; 2. If the tumour has a homogenous echo inside with a regional echoless zone, this is a reminder of the internal degeneration, such as bleeding, necrosis or cystic change; 3. In cases where the brachial plexus schwannoma that grows towards the inner side clings wholly or partly to the anterior scalene muscle, it can be judged that the tumour occurs at the root or trunk of the brachial plexus. 4. In cases where the brachial plexus schwannoma that grows towards the outer side partly

clings to the lateral and posterior anterior scalene muscle, the lesion is often misdiagnosed as a lymph node lesion.

4.1.4 Lesions of the Vagus Nerve, Phrenic Nerve and Accessory Nerve (Cases 21–22)

The vagus nerve, the longest and the most widely distributed cranial nerve, runs at the rear of the medulla oblongata olive below the filamentous glossopharyngeal nerve root, into the brain, and travels out of the cranial cavity through the jugular vein, downwards in the rear between the common carotid artery and the internal jugular vein in the neck. It then runs into the thoracic cavity through the superior opening of the thorax. The left vagus nerve runs between the left common carotid artery and the left subclavian artery and then descends to the front of the aortic arch. The right vagus nerve runs in front of the right subclavian artery and descends along the right side of the trachea.

The phrenic nerve, an important branch of the cervical plexus, generally begins from the C3–C5 nerve roots branching into the right phrenic nerve and the left phrenic nerve. The phrenic nerve descends to the inside, and along its front side is

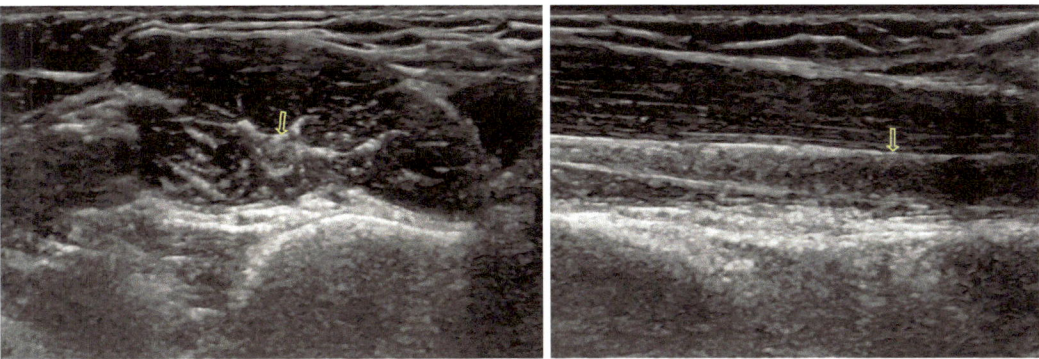

Fig. 4.31 Cord level injury (musculocutaneous nerve) of the brachial plexus. Note: the arrow is pointing to the short and long axes of the cord level injury (musculocutaneous nerve) of the brachial plexus

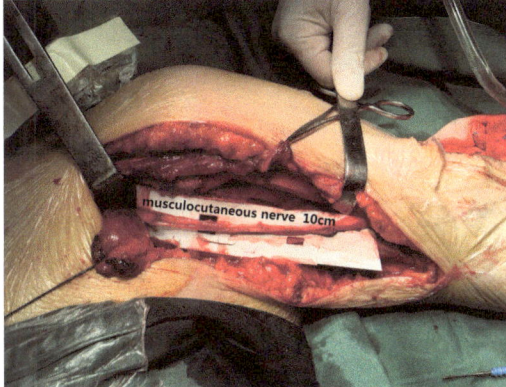

Fig. 4.32 Image of the operation for cord level injury (musculocutaneous nerve) of the brachial plexus

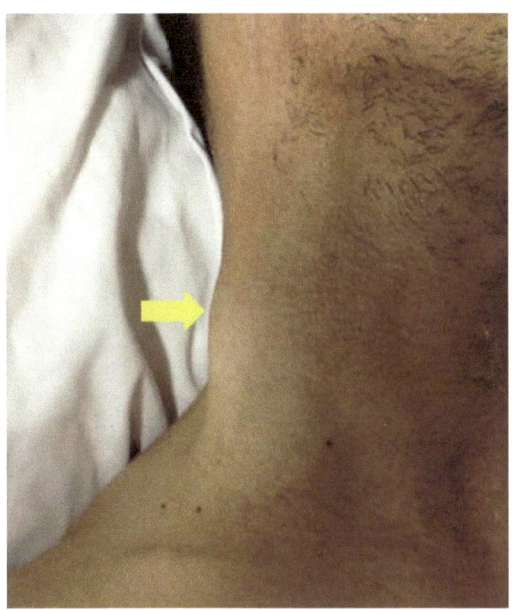

Fig. 4.33 External view of C7 neurilemmoma of the brachial plexus. Note: the yellow arrow indicates the mass

the superior end of the anterior scalene muscle. In all, 97% of phrenic nerve\branches enter the thoracic cavity through the superior opening of the thorax between the subclavian artery and vein, while the remaining 3% run in front of the subclavian vein.

The cranial root and spinal root nerve fuse and grow together to form the accessory nerve, which runs with the vagus nerve out of the cranial cavity from the jugular foramen, where it branches into two branches: the lateral branch and the medial branch. The lateral branch, mainly composed of a motor nerve, with its fibres coming from the C1–C3 cervical nerve roots, runs on the deep surface of

the sternocleidomastoid muscle and the superficial surface of the levator scapulae muscle, which makes it susceptible to iatrogenic injuries. Injuries may result as complications of routine surgical procedures such as cervical lymph node dissection, lymph node biopsy and jugular vein catheterization, with pain, muscle rigidity and dropped shoulder syndrome as clinical manifestations.

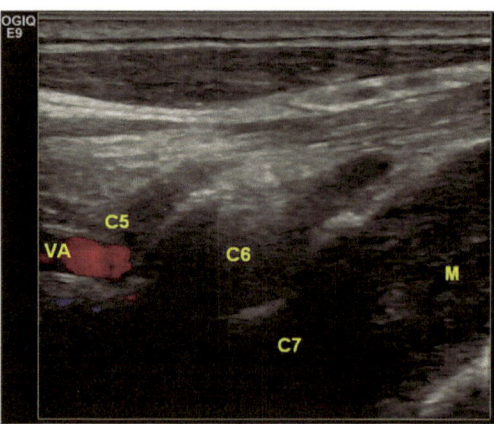

Fig. 4.34 Ultrasonogram of a C7 neurilemmoma of the brachial plexus. Note: C5 and C6 are normal nerve roots, M is the neurilemmoma from the C7 nerve root, and VA is the vertebral artery

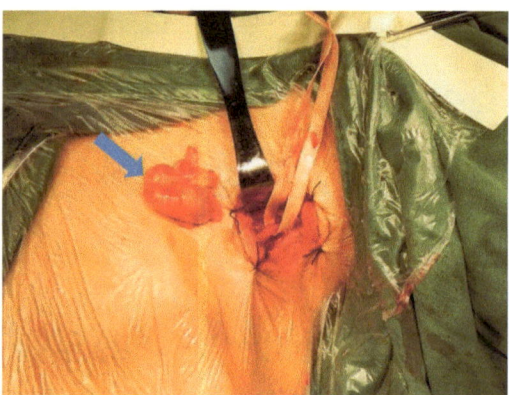

Fig. 4.36 Image of the operation for a C7 neurilemmoma of the brachial plexus. Note: the blue arrow indicates the excised neurilemmoma

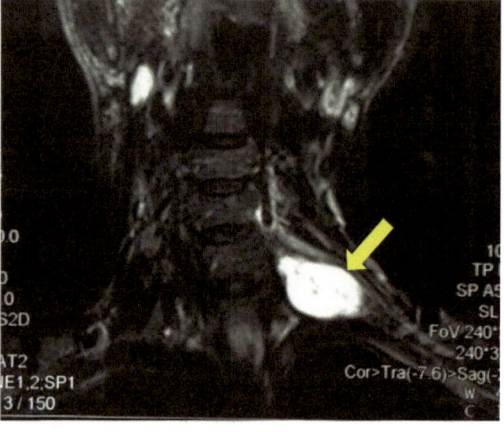

Fig. 4.35 MRI of a C7 neurilemmoma of the brachial plexus. Note: the yellow arrow indicates the C7 neurilemmoma

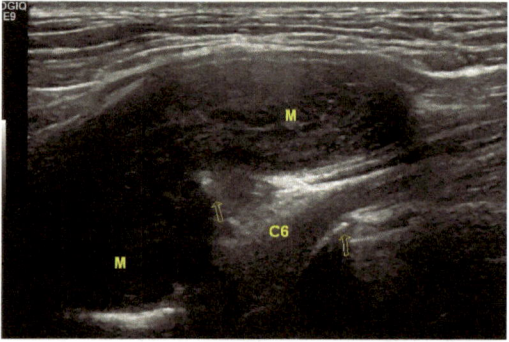

Fig. 4.37 Ultrasonogram of a C5 neurilemmoma of the brachial plexus. Note: the arrow indicates the transverse process of the cervical vertebra, C6 is a normal nerve, and M is the neurilemmoma from the C5 nerve root

Case 21

This case was a male patient, aged 34 years, with a cervical mass that was incidentally found during a physical examination. The ultrasound and MRI examinations at a local hospital led to a diagnosis of an enlarged cervical lymph gland. However, the ultrasonic examination at our hospital showed a cervical solid mass at the lateral common carotid artery. After further scans were performed, a lump was found connected with its surrounding nerves, presenting a rat tail sign. Therefore, this mass was diagnosed as a vagus nerve schwannoma, which was demonstrated by subsequent surgical pathol-

ogy (Figs. 4.52, 4.53, 4.54, 4.55, 4.56, 4.57, 4.58, 4.59 and 4.60) (Video 4.19).

ER 4.19 Dynamic image and explanation of a vagus nerve schwannoma

Case 22

See (Figs. 4.61 and 4.62) (Video 4.20).

ER 4.20 Dynamic image and explanation of vagus nerve neurofibromatosis

Summary In addition to the brachial plexus, the nerves in the neck also include the rarely seen accessory nerve, vagus nerve and phrenic nerve, which may also contain lesions.

Notes 1. During scanning of the phrenic nerve, the pressure on the probe should not be overly high, which would prevent neural compression leading to no ultrasonic display of lesions; 2. Accessory nerve injuries often occur after cervical lymph node biopsy, shouldering heavy things, cervical injuries and even massage, along with neural paralysis, and even nerve swelling and development of enlarged neuromas with a rhombic shape seen on local sections by ultrasonic examination; 3. For rare diseases such as vagus nerve lesions or vagus nerve neurofibroma, only by understanding the anatomical structures and routes of the above nerves can we make a correct diagnosis by ultrasound.

4.1.5 Cervical Plexus Lesions (Cases 23–24)

The cervical plexus consists of the anterior branches of the C1–C4 cervical nerves and is located in the deep part of the upper sternocleidomastoid in front of the middle scalene muscle and the levator scapulae muscle origin; the cervical plexus is divided into a superficial branch (skin branch) and a deep branch. The C1 nerve runs outwards to the upper and lower parts, the superior branches of the C2–C4 nerves run downwards from between the initial fibrous tissues of the anterior and middle scalene muscles and are divided into superior and inferior branches. The C1 and C2 superior branches merge together and then run in front of the neck, while the merged C2 superior branch and C3 inferior branch, together with the fused C3 inferior branch and the C4

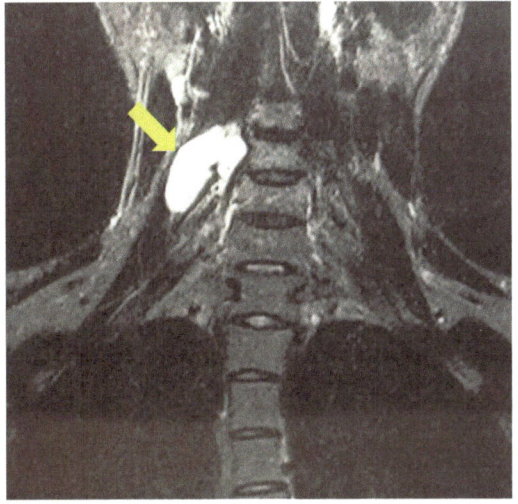

Fig. 4.38 MRI of a C5 neurilemmoma of the brachial plexus. Note: the yellow arrow indicates a C5 neurilemmoma

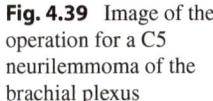
Fig. 4.39 Image of the operation for a C5 neurilemmoma of the brachial plexus

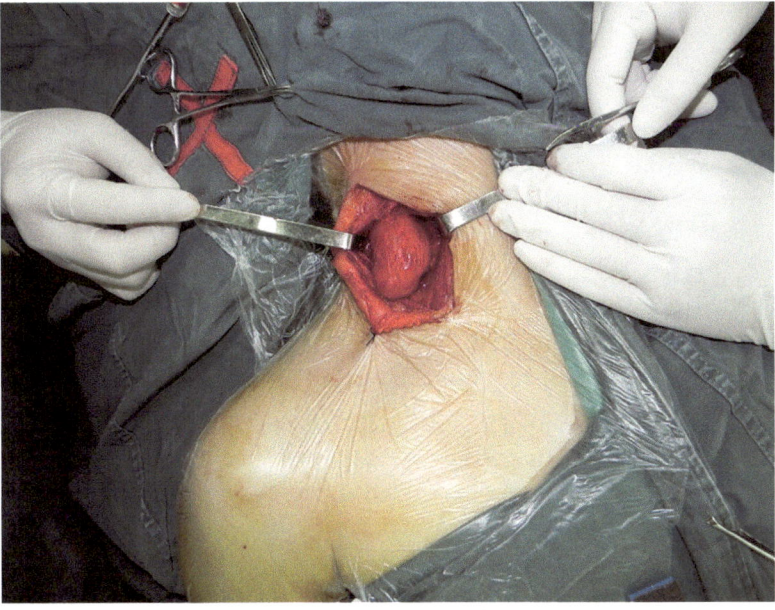

Fig. 4.40 Procedure chart of the excision of the neurilemmoma

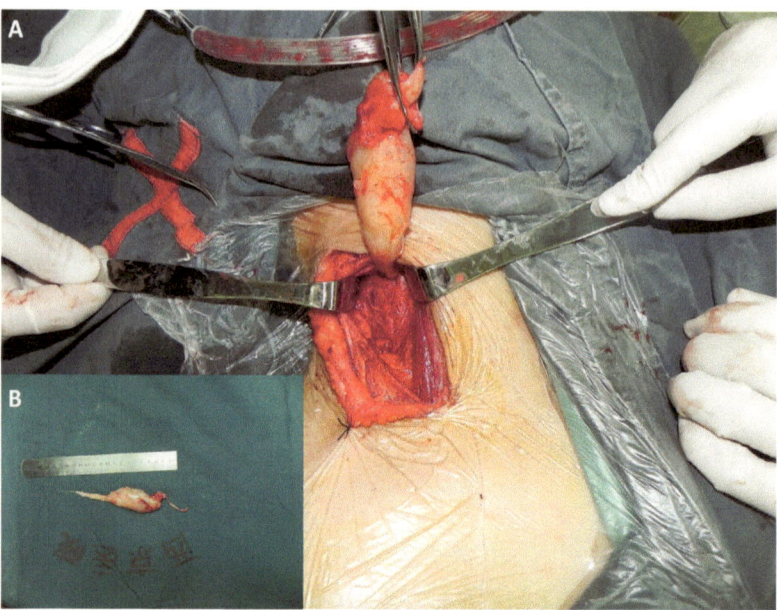

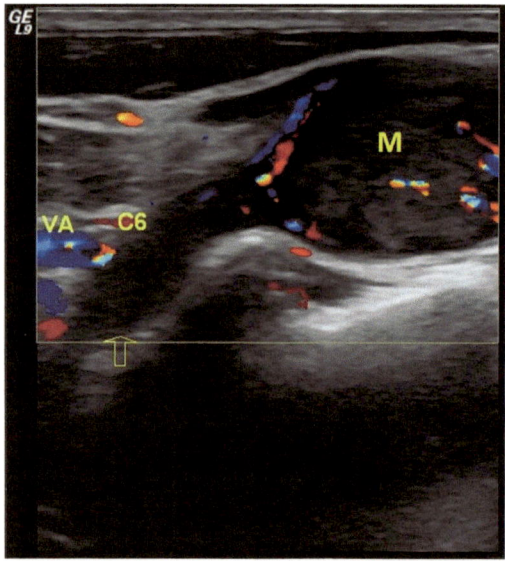

Fig. 4.41 Ultrasonogram of a C6 neurilemmoma of the brachial plexus. Note: the arrow indicates the C6 intervertebral foramen, VA is the vertebral artery and M is the C6 neurilemmoma

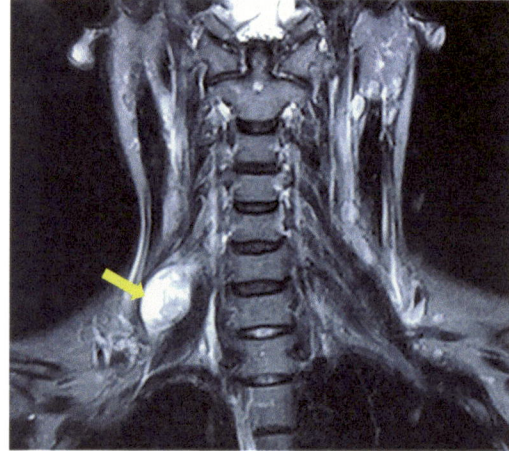

Fig. 4.42 MRI of a C6 neurilemmoma of the brachial plexus. Note: the yellow arrow indicates the C6 neurilemmoma

superior branch, run from the deep surface to the superficial surface. They then slant downwards through the cervical fascia tissues and split into 8–12 branches slightly above the midpoint of the rear edge of the sternocleidomastoid. The com-

mon symptoms of cervical plexus entrapment include shoulder pain. Cervical plexus block is a frequently used anaesthesia method, and familiarity with the cervical plexus anatomy is the basis of diagnosing cervical plexus lesions.

Case 23

A female patient, aged 28 years, had a right cervical mass that was found 6 years prior.

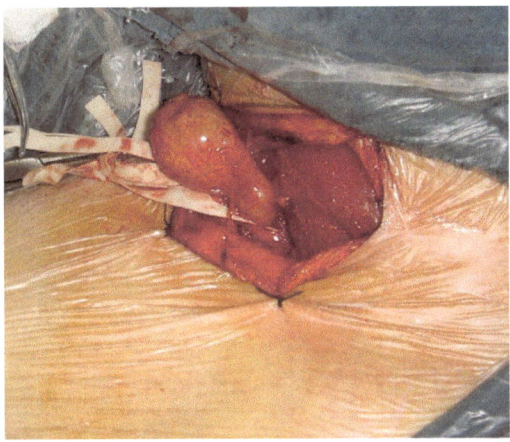

Fig. 4.43 Image of the operation for a C6 neurilemmoma of the brachial plexus

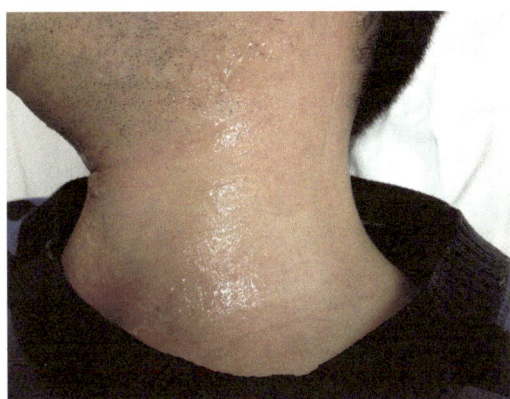

Fig. 4.45 External view of a C6 neurilemmoma of the brachial plexus

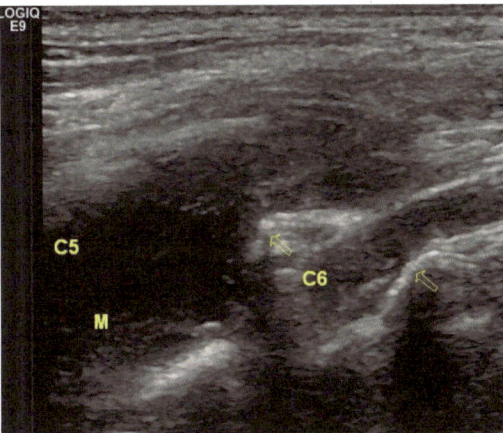

Fig. 4.44 Ultrasonogram of the cystic degeneration of a C5 neurilemmoma of the brachial plexus. Note: the arrow indicates the transverse process of the cervical vertebra, C6 is a normal nerve and M is the cystic degeneration of the C5 neurilemmoma

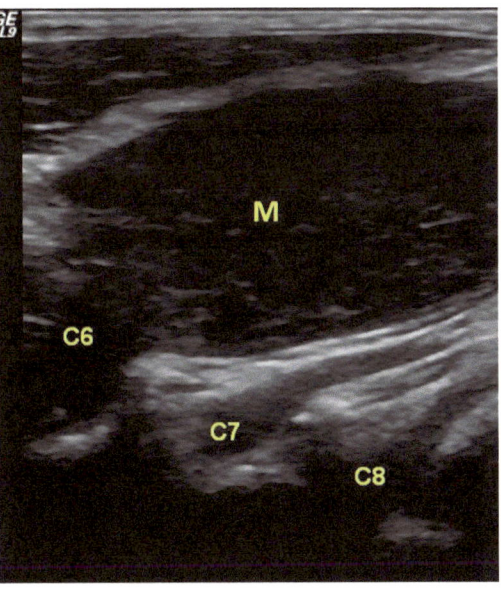

Fig. 4.46 Ultrasonogram of a C6 neurilemmoma of the brachial plexus. Note: C7 and C8 are normal nerves, and M is the neurilemmoma from the C6 nerve root

Current medical history: a mass approximately 2.0 × 3.0 cm was incidentally found in the right side of her neck; it was painful when pressed, with no obvious radiating pain, and no abnormities of skin sensation and motor functions. Thus, the patient received no special treatment. Recently, the patient presented at our hospital for diagnosis because the mass was enlarged and was painful upon palpation. MRI showed a cystic space-occupying lesion in the intervertebral foramen at the right C3-C5 centrum level. Therefore, a neurogenic tumour was considered.

Ultrasound: a solid hypoechoic mass 2.0 × 3.0 cm in the intervertebral foramen of the right C3 and C4 was growing outward with a blood supply inside; no obvious abnormalities in the brachial plexus were found. Therefore,

Fig. 4.47 Image of the operation for a C6 neurilemmoma of the brachial plexus

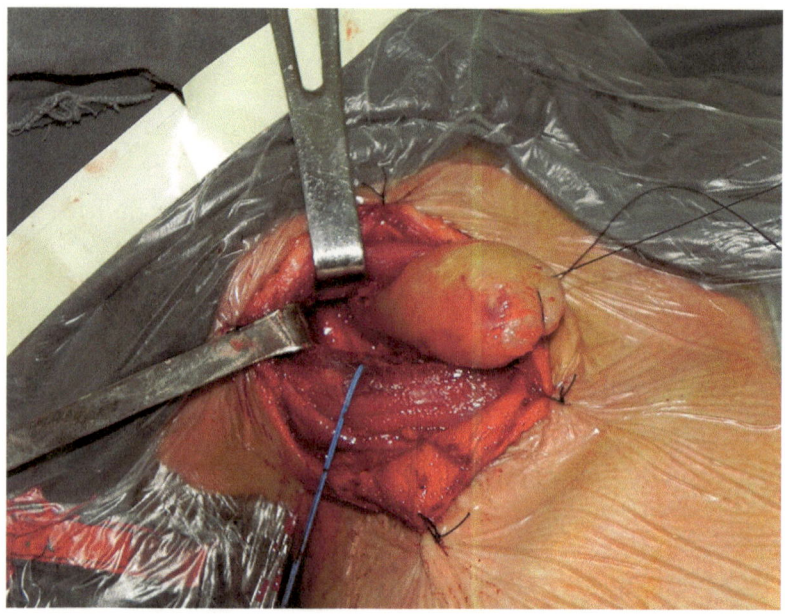

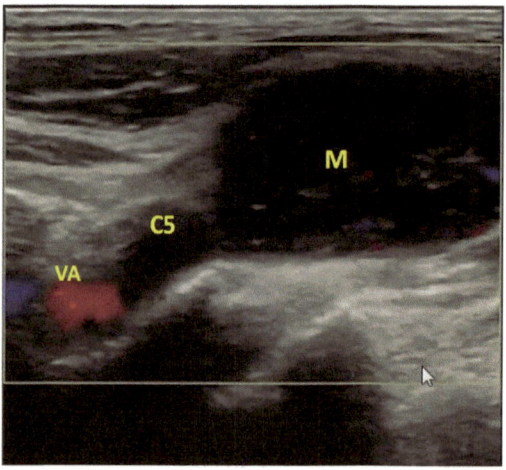

Fig. 4.48 Ultrasonogram of a C5 neurilemmoma of the brachial plexus. Note: M is the neurilemmoma from C5, and VA is the vertebral artery

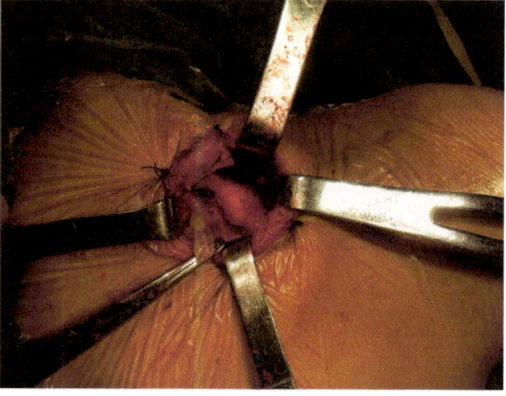

Fig. 4.49 Image of the operation for a C5 neurilemmoma of the brachial plexus

schwannoma of the cervical plexus was considered (Fig. 4.63) (Videos 4.21 and 4.22).

Operation: during surgery on the right neck, a mass was found at the deep surface of the sternocleidomastoid. After the mass was fully exposed and the sternocleidomastoid was moved aside, the mass was found to be covered by an intact membrane and had a clear boundary with the surrounding tissues. After separating the related great auricular nerve and accessory nerve for protection, and completely removing the mass, it was found that the 4.0 × 5.0 cm mass was greyish-brown in colour and was then diagnosed as a cervical plexus neural tumour after complete excision.

ER 4.21 Dynamic image and explanation of a cervical plexus C3 neuroma

ER4.22 Dynamic image of contrast-enhanced ultrasonography (CEUS) and explanation of a C3 neuroma of the cervical plexus

Case 24
See (Figs. 4.64 and 4.65).

Summary When patients experience cervical pain for unknown reasons, especially when a mass is found or when the limbs are numb, the doctor should consider scanning the cervical plexus, after brachial plexus injuries and lesions are ruled out, to identify enlarged lymph nodes and a metastatic tumour. Such patients generally present at the hospital after a physical examination, and they complain about dizziness and cervical discomfort, and then are often required to undergo CT and MRI examinations for intracranial structure to determine the initial clinical diagnosis. Therefore, the lesion is not easily found due to failure to examine the cervical plexus structure.

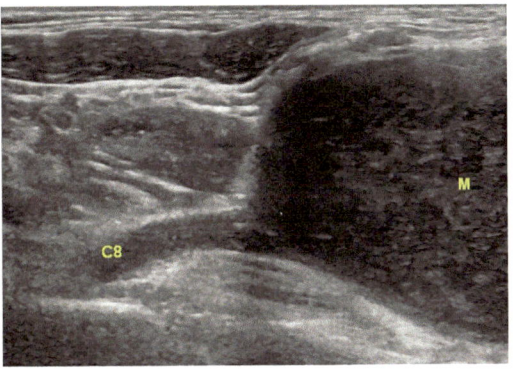

Fig. 4.50 Ultrasonogram of a C8 neurilemmoma of the brachial plexus. Note: M is the C8 neurilemmoma

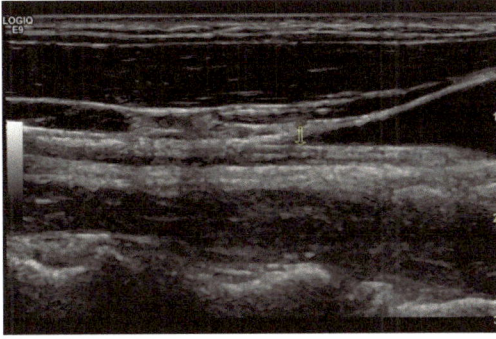

Fig. 4.52 Ultrasonogram of the long axis of normal vagus nerve. Note: the arrow indicates the vagus nerve

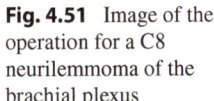

Fig. 4.51 Image of the operation for a C8 neurilemmoma of the brachial plexus

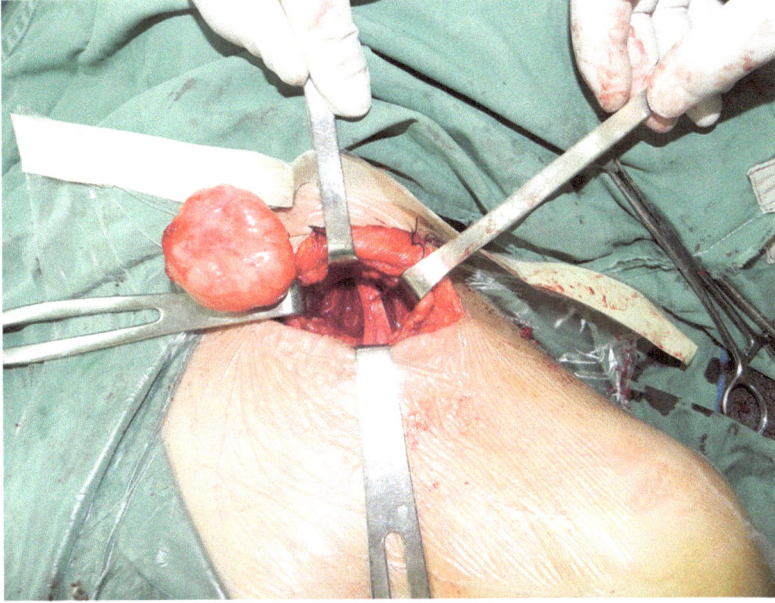

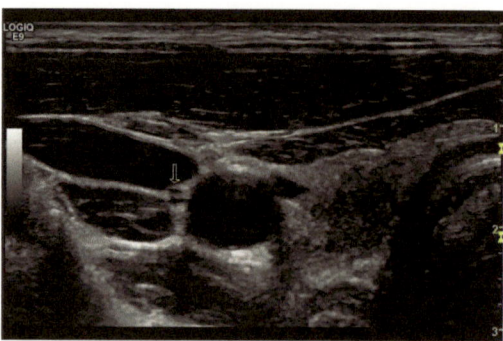

Fig. 4.53 Ultrasonogram of the short axis of normal vagus nerve. Note: the arrow indicates the vagus nerve

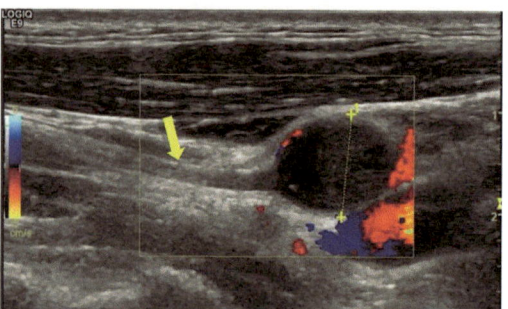

Fig. 4.54 Ultrasonogram of a vagus nerve schwannoma. Note: the yellow arrow indicates the vagus nerve, and the Vernier calliper indicates the schwannoma

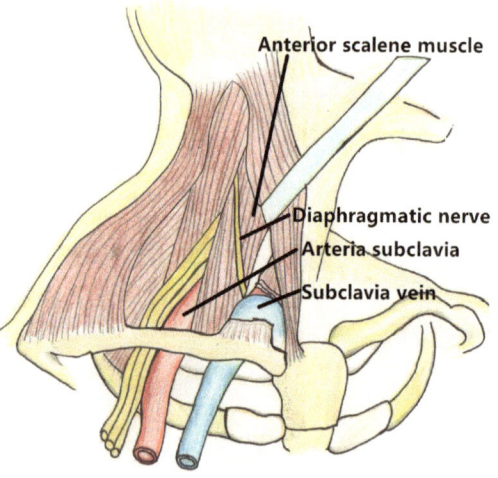

Fig. 4.55 Sketch map of a normal phrenic nerve

Anterior scalene muscle

Diaphragmatic nerve
Arteria subclavia
Subclavia vein

Notes 1. During examination, if no abnormity is found in the brachial plexus, the cervical plexus should be examined; 2. For patients with cervical

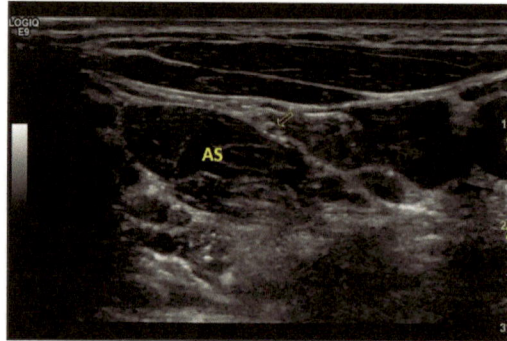

Fig. 4.56 Ultrasonogram of the short axis of a normal phrenic nerve. Note: AS is anterior scalene muscle and the arrow indicates the phrenic nerve

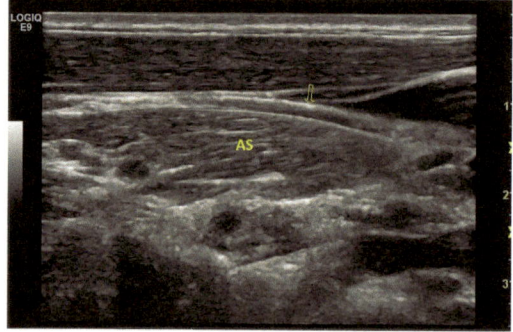

Fig. 4.57 Ultrasonogram of the long axis of a normal phrenic nerve. Note: AS is anterior scalene muscle and the arrow indicates the phrenic nerve

lumps or with pain upon palpation for a long time but without obvious lumps, the possibility of a high-position cervical plexus lesion should be considered, in addition to the common diseases caused by brachial plexus (entrapment).

4.2 Typical Cases of Neurological Diseases of the Upper Limb

Nerve entrapment may occur in any part of the path along which a nerve runs, but it is often seen at the fibrous or bone-fibre tunnels formed at bones or joints and the origin of tendons, ligaments and muscles. Nerves run through fixed anatomic sites in these potential pathways. The neural diseases that result from nerve entrapment due to the inflammatory thickening of ligament, muscle,

Fig. 4.58 Ultrasono-
gram and scanning
diagram of the short axis
of a normal accessory
nerve. Note: in (**a**), LSM
is the levator scapulae
muscle, and the arrow
indicates the short axis
of the accessory nerve;
(**b**) is the scan diagram
of the accessory nerve

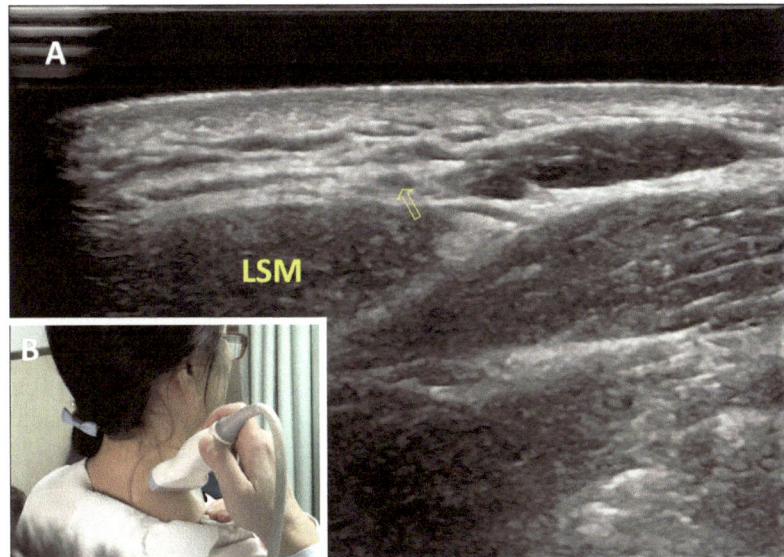

Fig. 4.59 Image of the
operation for accessory
nerve injury and its body
surface appearance.
Note: in (**a**), the yellow
arrow indicates the
accessory nerve injury,
and in (**b**), the yellow
arrow indicates the body
surface appearance
before surgery

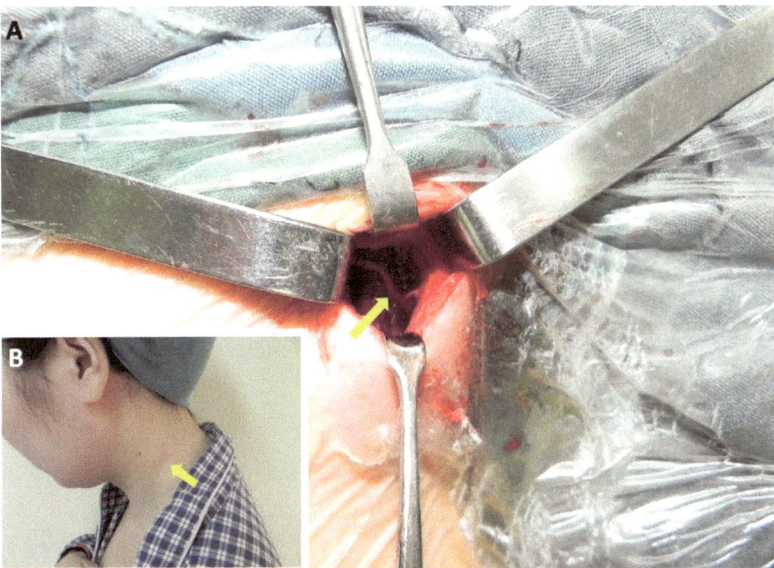

tendon, tendon sheath or synovial membrane, soft tissue space-occupying lesions (tumour, cyst or haematoma), bone abnormalities (fracture, bony spur, bony exostosis or bony callus), injuries caused by over exercising and occupational lesions, are commonly called nerve entrapment syndrome or nerve compression syndrome. In addition, compression by inflammation, tumour, cyst and haematoma of the structures parallel to nerves such as muscles, tendons and blood vessels and surrounding fibrous and fatty tissues is also included into such a syndrome. The common entrapment syndromes in the upper limbs include carpal tunnel syndrome, cubital tunnel syndrome and thoracic outlet syndrome. Their main ultrasonogram features are as follows: (1) In case of obvious entrapment, the local neural section becomes thin and is accompanied by reduced echo intensity, while the nerves at the proximal end or at both ends are enlarged with hypoechoic change; (2) When scar conglutination occurs, the epineurium and perineurium of enlarged nerves

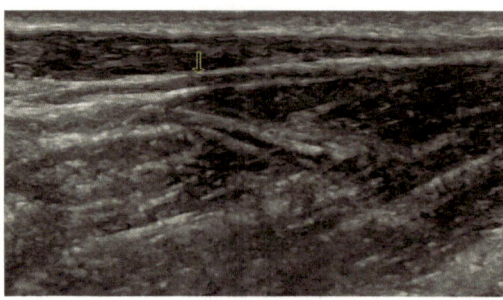

Fig. 4.60 Ultrasonogram of the long axis of an accessory nerve injury. Note: the arrow is pointing to the enlarged accessory nerve with oedema

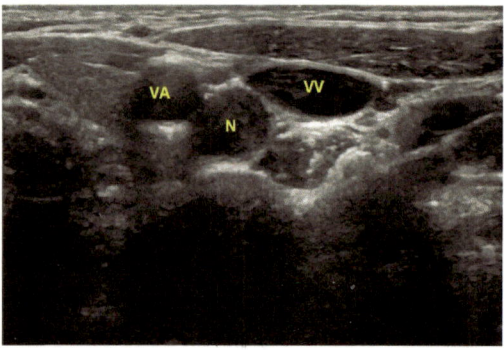

Fig. 4.61 Ultrasonogram of a vagus nerve neurofibroma. Note: *VA* carotid artery, *VV* jugular vein, *N* vagus nerve neurofibroma

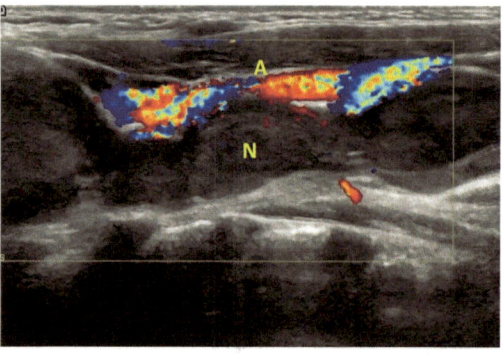

Fig. 4.62 Colour Doppler flow imaging of vagus nerve neurofibromatosis. Note: *N* vagus nerve neurofibromatosis, *A* carotid artery

usually present as a blurred bundle structure. In addition, the long-term and repetitive entrapment can cause tumour-like hyperplasia, which is another manifestation of nerve entrapment disorders.

4.2.1 Median Nerve Injury (Cases 25–30)

Median nerve entrapment syndrome can be divided into pronator teres muscle syndrome, interosseous palmar nerve compression syndrome and carpal tunnel syndrome according to different compression positions. The last one is commonly seen in women and primarily results from continuous increases in pressure in the carpal canal due to hyperplasia of soft tissues or reduced volume of the carpal canal. The main clinical indicators include a reduction in thumb, forefinger, middle finger, and radial ring finger skin sensation, accompanied by numbness and pain at night, which severely affects the patients' sleep quality. If such a disease is not treated, the thenar muscle may have amyotrophy, leading to inflexible thumbs and a reduction or loss of grabbing ability, which thus significantly affects patients' work and daily lives [3, 4].

Case 25

A male patient, aged 56 years, experienced gout for over 10 years. Main complaint: numbness of his right forearm and resistance of right hand extension-flexion for over 10 months. Physical examination: the pathway of median nerve at his right wrist presented Tinel's sign (+), the right wrist presented flexion and was unable to be stretched; his right thumb was unable to bend towards the palm, and presented OK sign (+); he also had weakness when opening and closing the fingers and the clipping paper test presented (+). His right palm and fingers were numb below the wrist crease, his right radial artery pulse was weak, and the temperature at the distal ends of his fingers was lower than that at the uninjured side.

Ultrasonic examination: the right median nerve ran continuously, but the local nerve was 1.88 cm × 0.42 cm in size at the wrist, and as the scanning continued, it was observed to be enlarged with a cross-sectional area of 0.56 cm². Ultrasound finding: median nerve injury at the right wrist along with entrapment (Figs. 4.66, 4.67, 4.68 and 4.69) (Video 4.23).

Operation: after incision of the carpal canal from the carpal canal distal end level to the median

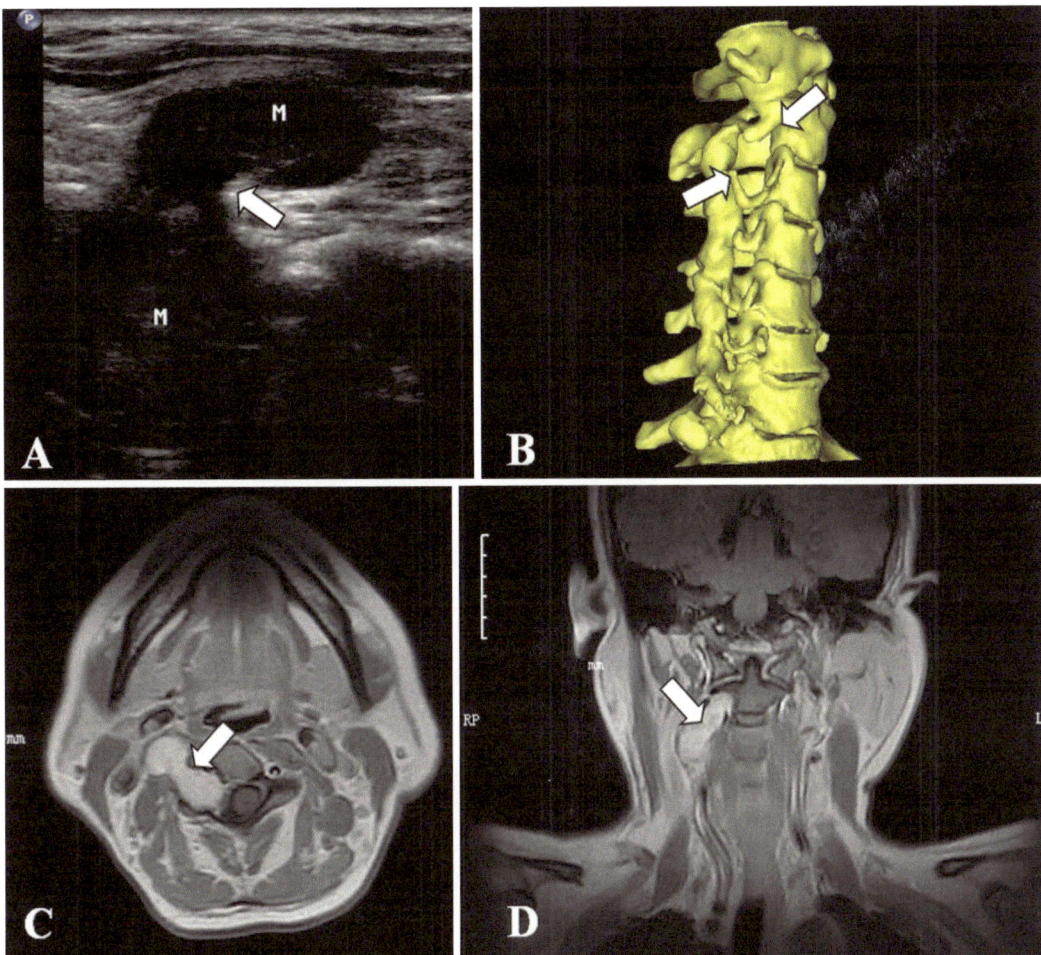

Fig. 4.63 C3 neural tumour of the cervical plexus. Note: in (**a**), the arrow is pointing to the transverse process of the vertebra and M is the neuroma lesion from the intervertebral foramen; in (**b**), the arrow is pointing to the enlarged intervertebral foramen by 3D-reconstruction; in (**c**), the arrow is pointing to the lesion growing outwards from the intervertebral foramen in an MRI cross section; in (**d**), the arrow is pointing to the lesion growing outwards from the intervertebral foramen in an MRI longitudinal section

nerve distal end, a thickened transverse ligament of the wrist was found. After incising it to loosen and wash the median nerve, the nerve's continuity was still preserved, but a 2-cm section was enlarged at the wrist crease level, and its nerve tract appeared tawny.

ER 4.23 Dynamic image and explanation of the gout-induced median nerve compression of the carpal canal

Case 26
See (Figs. 4.70 and 4.71) (Videos 4.24 and 4.25).

ER 4.24 Dynamic image and explanation of carpal tunnel syndrome

ER 4.25 Explanation of carpal tunnel syndrome during surgery

Case 27
A female patient aged 44 years. Main complaint: the left radial three and half fingers were numb for over 3 months due to injury. Current medical history: the patient immediately experienced pain, bleeding, finger numbness and confined movements followed by left wrist injury 3 months

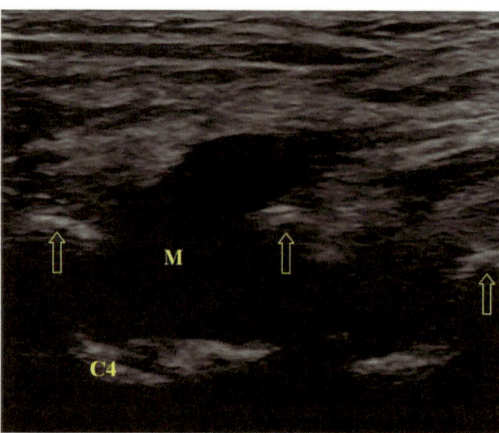

Fig. 4.64 Ultrasonogram of a neuroma in the C4 cervical plexus. Note: the arrow is pointing to the transverse process, and M is the neural lesion from the intervertebral foramen

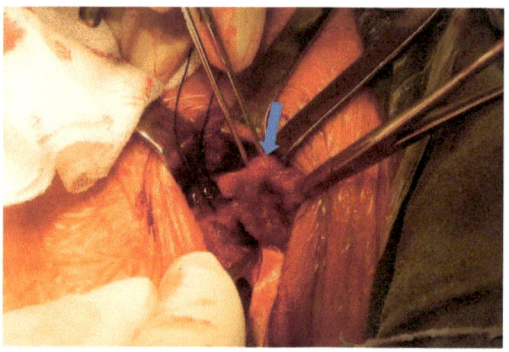

Fig. 4.65 Image of the operation for a neuroma in the C4 cervical plexus. Note: the blue arrow is pointing to the neural lesion

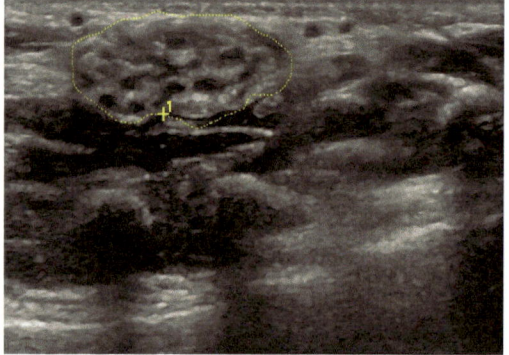

Fig. 4.66 Ultrasonogram (short axis) of gout-induced median nerve entrapment of the carpal canal. Note: the dashed line beside the calliper indicates the enlarged median nerve cross section with oedema

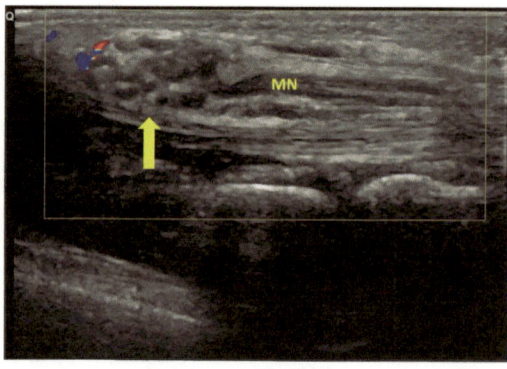

Fig. 4.67 Ultrasonogram (long axis) of gout-induced median nerve entrapment of the carpal canal. Note: MN is median nerve, and the yellow arrow is pointing to the enlarged median nerve with oedema

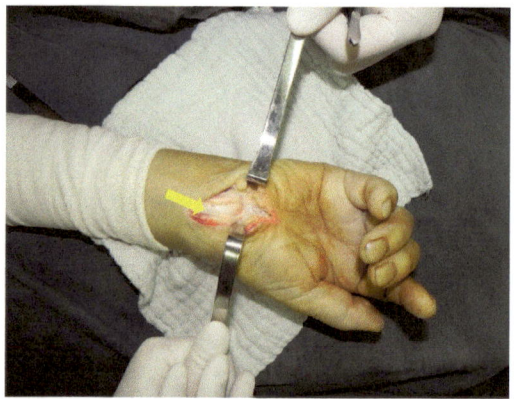

Fig. 4.68 Picture of the operation for gout-induced median nerve entrapment of the carpal canal (before loosening the median nerve). Note: the yellow arrow is pointing to the enlarged carpal canal median nerve with oedema

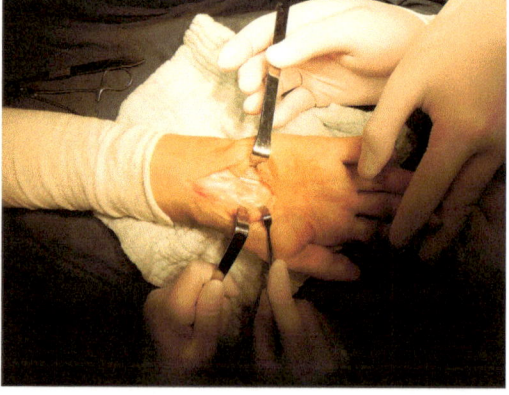

Fig. 4.69 Image of the operation for gout-induced median nerve entrapment of the carpal canal (after loosening the median nerve)

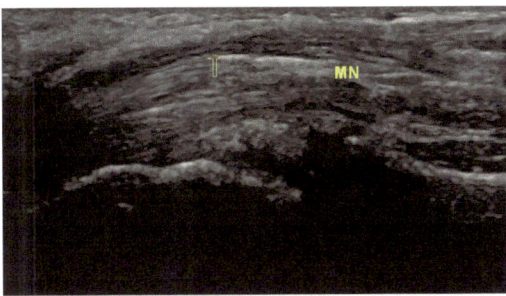

Fig. 4.70 Ultrasonogram of median nerve entrapment of the cubital tunnel. Note: MN is median nerve, and the arrow is pointing to oedema of the median nerve

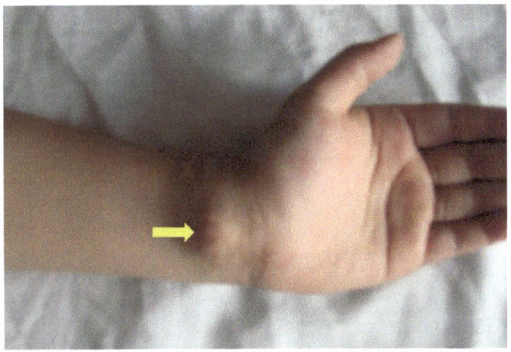

Fig. 4.72 External view of a traumatic neuroma of the median nerve. Note: the yellow arrow is pointing to the superficial lump

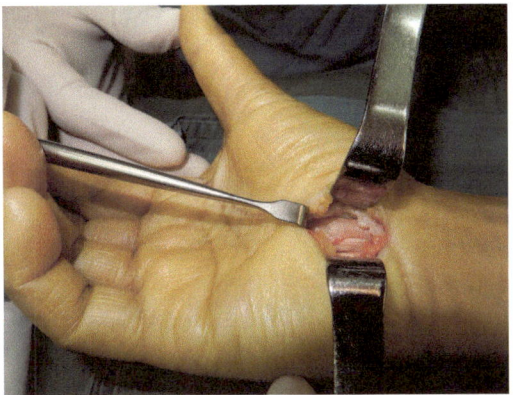

Fig. 4.71 Image of the operation for median nerve release. Note: the arrow is pointing to the median nerve

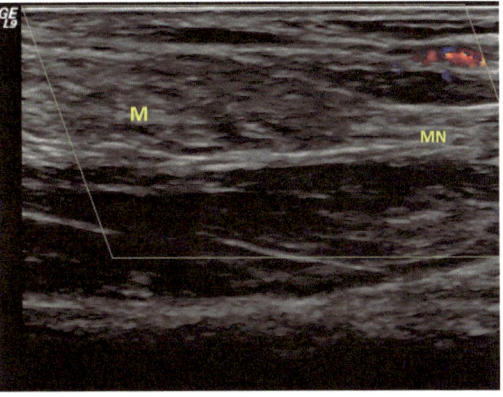

Fig. 4.73 Ultrasonogram of a traumatic neuroma of the median nerve. Note: *MN* median nerve and M: the traumatic neuroma of the median nerve

prior; she then went to a local hospital for neural debridement at the left wrist as well as for tendon examination and repair before an external plaster fixation operation. After 1 month, when the plaster was removed, the patient performed active and passive exercises, but the numbness remained. Specialized physical examination: a U-shaped injury and surgical scar were observed at the left wrist, with slight atrophy of the left thenar eminence muscle. The acupuncture sensation for the three and a half fingers at the radial side of the left hand was reduced, while the other one and a half fingers at the ulnar side had no abnormities. The scar at the left wrist had Tinel's sign (+).

Ultrasound: the median nerve at the left wrist was not shown clearly on ultrasound, and on the deep surface of the scar, a hypoechoic zone approximately 1.5 cm × 0.6 cm in size with an irregular form was observed, as was a blurred boundary with the surrounding tissues. Its distal end diameter measured 0.29 cm, while the proximal end measured 0.30 cm. Tip: the hypoechoic zone near the scar at the left wrist was considered a median nerve injury in addition to a scar neuroma (Figs. 4.72, 4.73 and 4.74) (Video 4.26).

Operation: during surgery, it was found that large amounts of scar tissue had formed and demonstrated severe adhesion to the median nerve and muscle tendon controlling finger flexion. It was necessary to thoroughly loosen the muscle tendon, especially since the neural muscle tendon had been sutured. The transverse ligament of the wrist was vertically incised to loosen the median nerve. Postoperative diagnosis: traumatic neuroma of the left median nerve.

ER 4.26 Dynamic image and explanation of traumatic neuroma of the median nerve

Case 28
See (Figs. 4.75 and 4.76) (Videos 4.27 and 4.28).

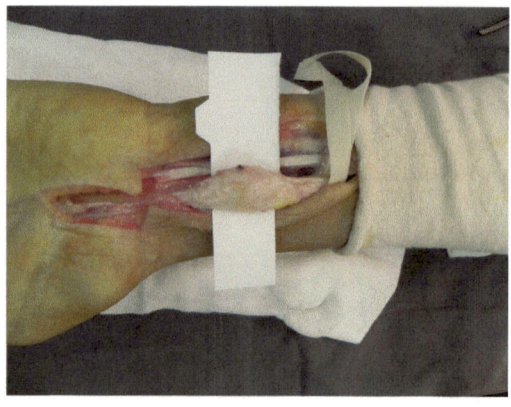

Fig. 4.74 Image of the operation for traumatic neuroma of the median nerve

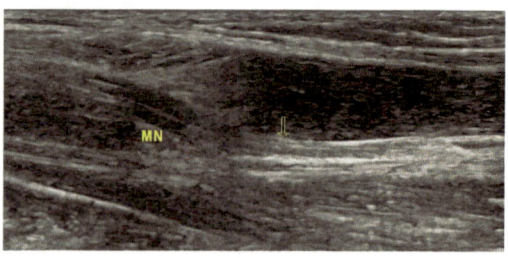

Fig. 4.75 Ultrasonogram of a lipoma enveloping the median nerve. Note: the arrow is pointing to the median nerve; the hyperechoic zone around the median nerve is the lipoma

ER 4.27 Dynamic image and explanation of a lipoma enveloping the median nerve

ER 4.28 Explanation of a lipoma enveloping the median nerve during surgery

Case 29
See (Fig. 4.77) (Video 4.29).

ER 4.29 Dynamic image and explanation of a median nerve injury at the axilla in the upper arm

Case 30
See (Figs. 4.78, 4.79, 4.80 and 4.81) (Video 4.30).

ER 4.30 Dynamic image and explanation of a fracture of the median nerve and radial nerve

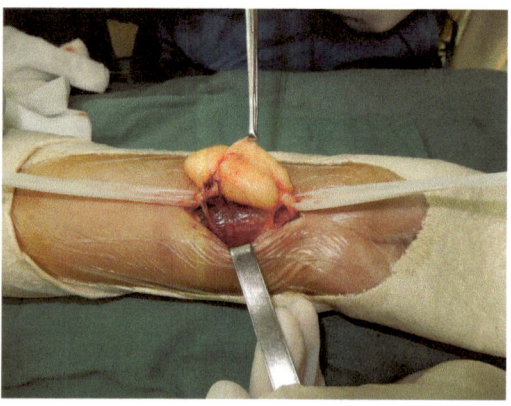

Fig. 4.76 Image of a lipoma enveloping the median nerve during surgery

Fig. 4.77 Ultrasonogram of a median nerve injury at the axilla. Note: in (**a**), M is the median nerve injury; in (**b**), the yellow arrow is pointing to the enlarged median nerve at the axilla, and the formation of neuroma

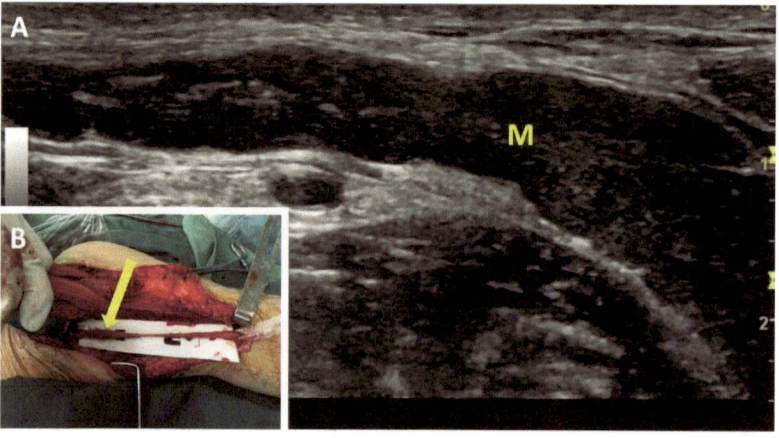

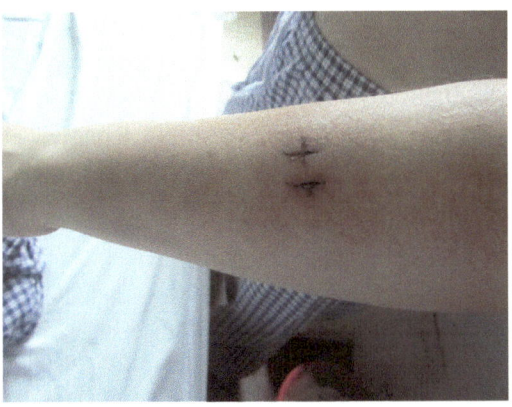

Fig. 4.78 External view of fractures of the median nerve and radial nerve

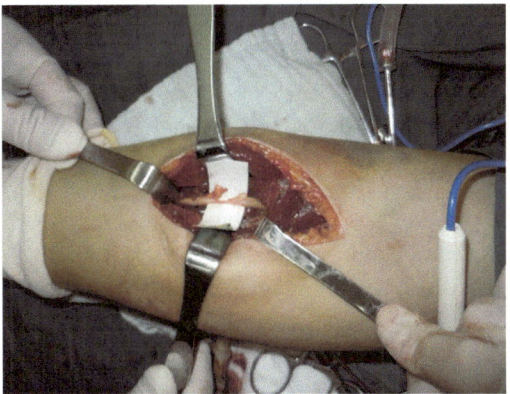

Fig. 4.80 Image of the operation for median nerve fracture (before suture)

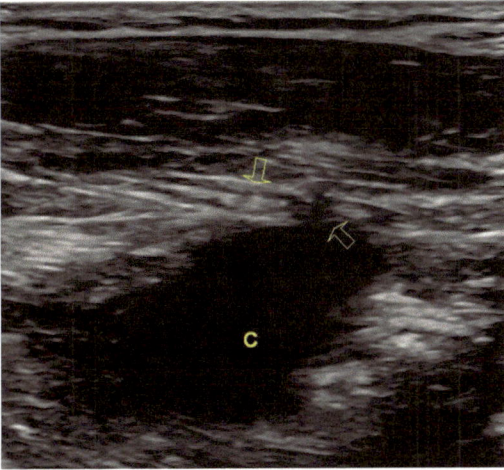

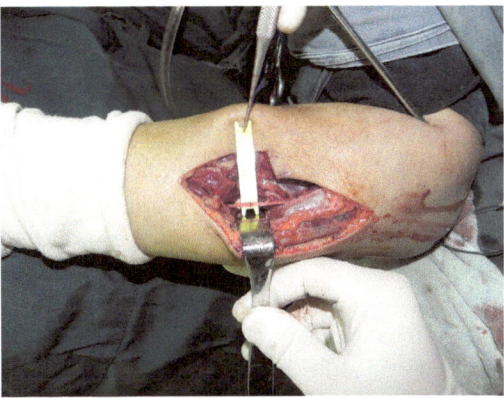

Fig. 4.81 Image of the operation for median nerve fracture (after suture)

Fig. 4.79 Ultrasonogram of a median nerve fracture. Note: the arrow is pointing to the location of the neural fracture, and C is haematoma

Summary 1. Median nerve injury often has indicators of carpal tunnel syndrome and trauma-induced neuroma in most cases; 2. In cases where median nerve injury is confirmed clinically but when the injury level is difficult to determine, scanning should strictly follow the anatomical structure of the median nerve, ulnar nerve and radial nerve; 3. In cases where the typical symptoms of median nerve injury emerge and no lesions are present in the forearms, scanning should move upwards towards the level of the axilla to find any lesions, thus preventing a missed diagnosis; 4. During ultrasonic examination, the probe should be vertical to the muscle tendon controlling finger flexion; otherwise, the tendon's echo may change, and it would be more difficult to differentiate the median nerve from the flexor tendon [5, 6].

4.2.2 Ulnar Nerve Injury (Cases 31–35)

Injuries to the ulnar nerve located in the superficial position in the cubital tunnel are closely associated with the anatomical structure of the nerve. Lesions behind the elbows, such as soft tissue thickening, bone dislocation, blood vessels that cross nerves, a mass and repeated elbow flexion, can compress the ulnar nerve, thereby causing cubital tunnel syndrome. The clinical indicators of cubital tunnel syndrome include numbness of the ring finger and litter finger, weakening and disappearance of sensation, poor fine motor movements of the hands and atrophy of some of the muscles. By physical examination, elbow flexion and Tinel's sign are positive. The ultrasonic results show that the nerve at the entrapment site is crooked and becomes thin. The proximal neural section is enlarged and oedematous; the neural bundle structure vanishes and presents a low echo. In severe cases, a pseudo-neuroma might develop [7–9].

Case 31

A female patient aged 46 years. Main complaint: the ulnar ring finger and little finger of her right hand were numb for 4 months since she sustained a right elbow injury. Current medical history: the patient's ulnar ring finger and little finger of her right hand were severely numb after she accidentally hit her right elbow on a tea table 4 months prior. However, no obvious wounds or traumatic bleeding of her elbow occurred, and thus the patient did not visit a hospital for diagnosis and treatment. Over the past 4 months, her symptoms remained; even the power and flexibility of her right hand had become weak, with her right ring finger and little finger unable to stretch to a straight position. Specialized physical examination: no obvious deformation of her right elbow was observed, but a stripe-like variation could be felt on her cubital ulnar nerve; the ulnar side of her right hand, the hypothenar muscle, little finger and half of her ring finger experienced hypaesthesia, with unobvious interosseous muscle atrophy of the right hypothenar muscle. Her little finger and ring finger appeared to be slightly claw-shaped, and Tinel's sign at the ulnar nerve groove was positive. Electromyogram: electrophysiologic manifestation of a medium-severe injury of the ulnar nerve at the right elbow.

Ultrasonic examination: it was found that the cubital ulnar nerve ran smoothly with its distal neural section narrowing to 0.20 cm in diameter. The partial proximal neural section had a tumour-like stripe-shaped variation and was enlarged to 1.0 cm in length, 0.35 cm in thickness and 0.16 cm^2 in cross-sectional area. Ultrasonic examination: ulnar nerve injury (entrapment) at the right elbow, with neuroma formation (Figs. 4.82, 4.83 and 4.84) (Video 4.31).

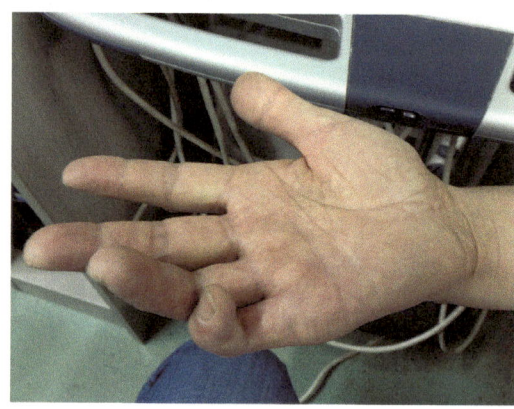

Fig. 4.82 External view of ulnar nerve entrapment in cubital tunnel syndrome (claw-hand)

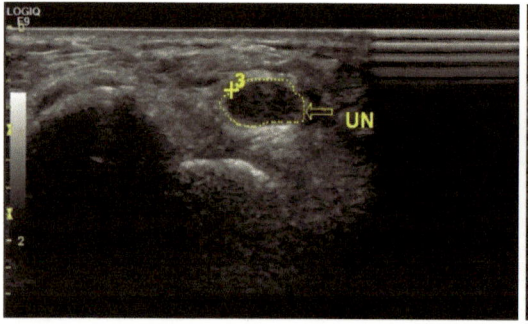

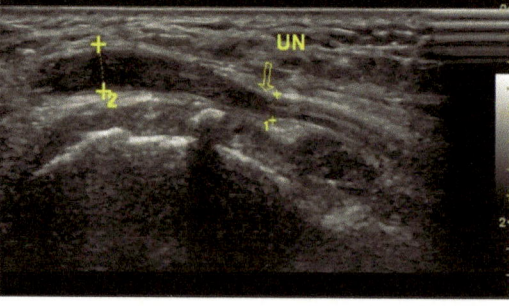

Fig. 4.83 Ultrasonogram of ulnar nerve entrapment in cubital tunnel syndrome. Note: UN is the short and long axes of the ulnar nerve, the dotted line beside the Vernier calliper in the left figure is the cross-sectional area of the ulnar nerve, and the arrow in the right figure is pointing to the narrowed ulnar nerve due to entrapment

Operation: the ulnar nerve at the right elbow ran continuously but was compressed at the cubital tunnel. After incising the cubital tunnel and freeing the ulnar nerve, part of the nerve was enlarged, and degeneration and a stripe-shaped tumour-like variation were also observed. Postoperative diagnosis: ulnar nerve entrapment at the right elbow.

ER 4.31 Dynamic image and explanation of ulnar nerve compression in cubital tunnel syndrome

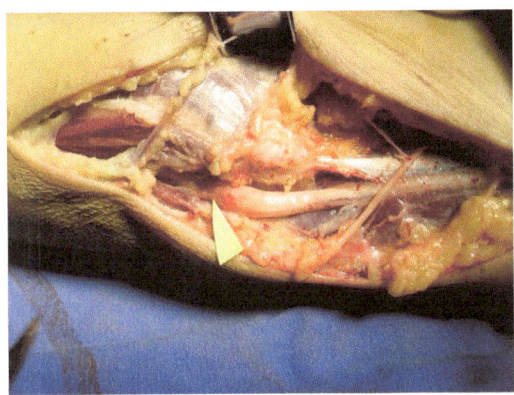

Fig. 4.84 Image of the operation for ulnar nerve entrapment in cubital tunnel syndrome. Note: the arrow is pointing to the location of ulnar nerve entrapment

Case 32
See (Fig. 4.85).

Case 33
See (Figs. 4.86 and 4.87).

Case 34
See (Figs. 4.88, 4.89 and 4.90).

Case 35
See (Figs. 4.91 and 4.92).

Summary Limb pain, numbness or functional obstacles caused by chronic entrapment or injuries resulting from peripheral nerve compression are commonly seen in clinical examination (such as carpal tunnel syndrome and cubital tunnel syndrome). Early diagnosis is conducive to selecting optimum treatment timing and modalities for eliminating entrapment and improving neural microcirculation as soon as possible. This would promote regeneration of the myelin sheath, prevent irreversible changes, and restore neural functions as early as possible.

Notes 1. Prior to scanning, knowledge of the patient's medical history and physical signs is helpful for the examination of neural injuries and lesions; 2. Attention should be paid to the nerve's

Fig. 4.85 Ultrasonogram of ulnar nerve entrapment in cubital tunnel syndrome. Note: *UN* ulnar nerve, the dotted line beside the Vernier calliper is the cross-sectional area of the ulnar nerve, and the arrow in the right figure is pointing to the location of ulnar nerve entrapment

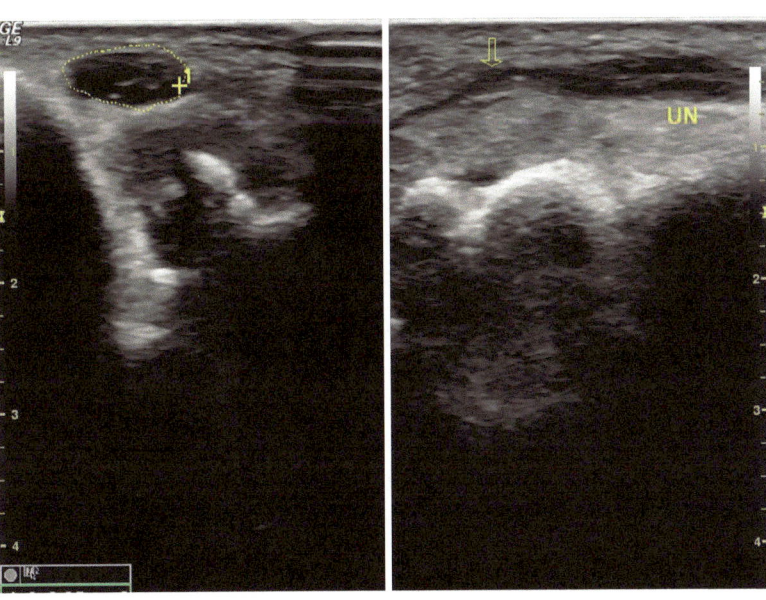

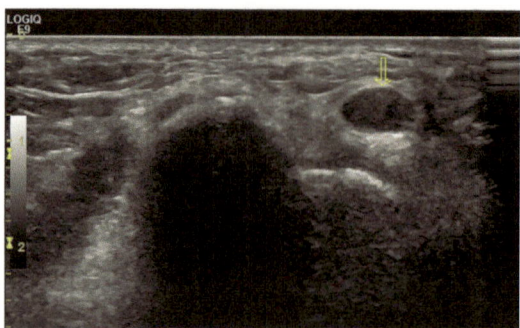 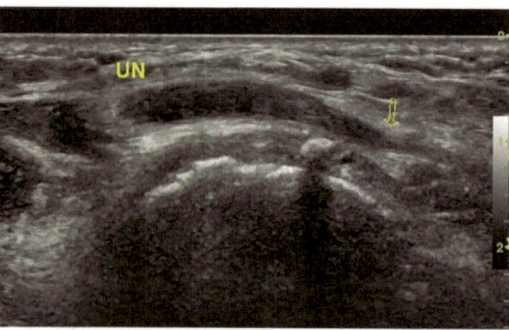

Fig. 4.86 Ultrasonogram of ulnar nerve entrapment in cubital tunnel syndrome. Note: *UN* ulnar nerve, the arrow in the left figure is the short axis of the ulnar nerve, and the

arrow in the right figure is pointing to the location of ulnar nerve entrapment

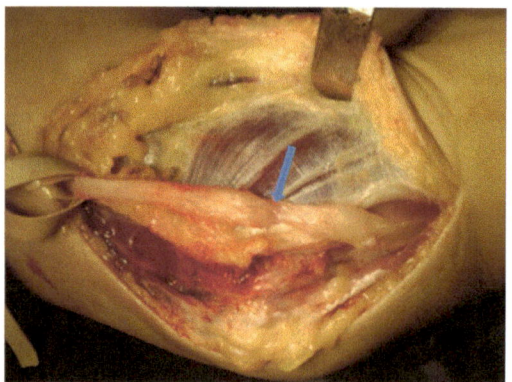 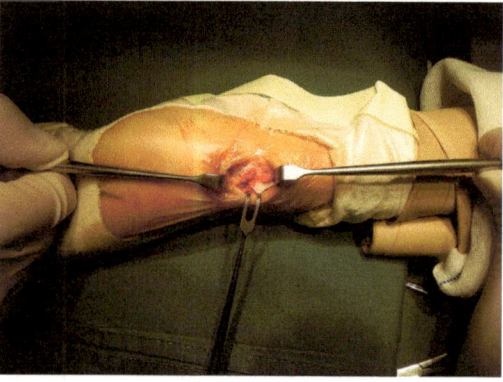

Fig. 4.87 Image of the operation for ulnar nerve entrapment in cubital tunnel syndrome. Note: the blue arrow is pointing to the location of ulnar nerve entrapment

Fig. 4.89 Image of the operation for ulnar nerve fracture (before suture)

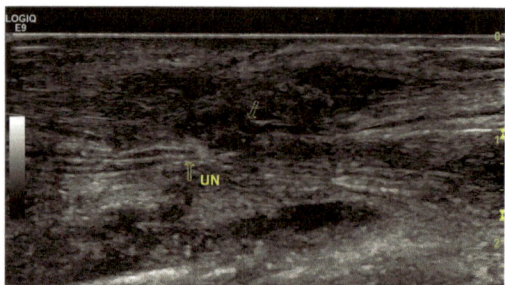 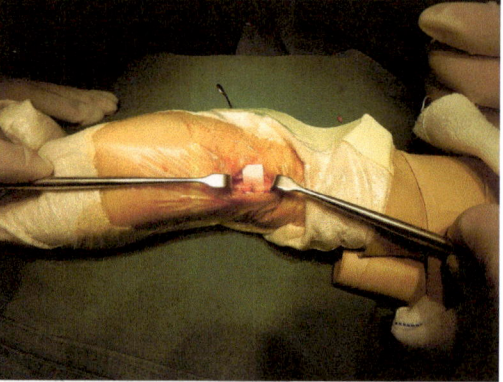

Fig. 4.88 Ultrasonogram of a fracture of the ulnar nerve. Note: *UN* ulnar nerve, and the arrow is pointing to a fracture of the ulnar nerve

Fig. 4.90 Image of the operation for ulnar nerve fracture (after suture)

path, the injury position and the change in its diameter, and the continuity of the injured nerve's path and its recovery after anastomosis should be observed; 3. Observe the completeness of the neural structure on cross section as well as the

continuity of its bundle structure on its longitudinal section to judge the degree of neural injury due to entrapment.

4.2.3 Ulnar Nerve Mutation (Absence) (Case 36)

Ulnar nerve mutation: In cases of ulnar nerve mutation, the ulnar nerve is not located in the ulnar nerve groove, but rather, in front of the epicondyle in the humerus. Since the ulnar nerve groove is unable to confine the ulnar nerve, the ulnar nerve will experience friction with the surrounding tissues with the movement of joints, thereby leading to neuritis and even occasional cases of ulnar nerve absence.

Case 36
See (Figs. 4.93, 4.94, 4.95 and 4.96) (Videos 4.32 and 4.33).

ER 4.32 Dynamic image and explanation of absence of the ulnar nerve

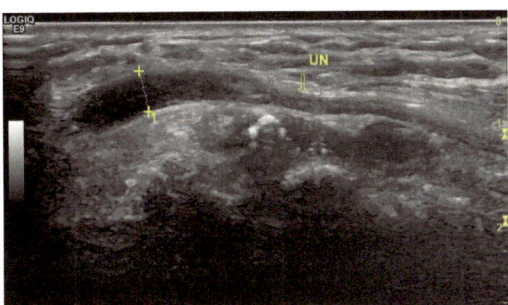

Fig. 4.91 Ultrasonogram for ulnar nerve entrapment in cubital tunnel syndrome (formation of neuroma). Note: *UN* ulnar nerve, the arrow is pointing to the location of ulnar nerve entrapment, and the Vernier calliper indicates the formation of an ulnar nerve neuroma

ER 4.33 Dynamic image and explanation of normal contralateral ulnar nerve in a patient with ulnar nerve absence

Summary 1. The patient has typical symptoms of ulnar nerve injury. When obvious muscular atrophy can be seen in the limbs, the ulnar nerve's path should be scanned first; 2. When abnormalities are found, the contralateral ulnar nerve should be compared with the injured nerve by scanning in order to correctly diagnose the patient.

4.2.4 Neural Cyst Entrapment (Cases 37–42)

Neural entrapment due to cysts inside and outside a nerve is a clinically rare peripheral nerve disorder. Ultrasound intuitively confirms the form, path and position of a nerve entrapment injury and identifies

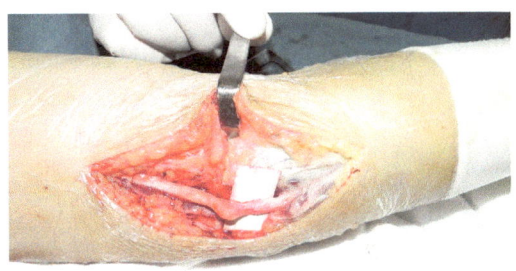

Fig. 4.92 Image of the operation for ulnar nerve entrapment in cubital tunnel syndrome (neuroma formed)

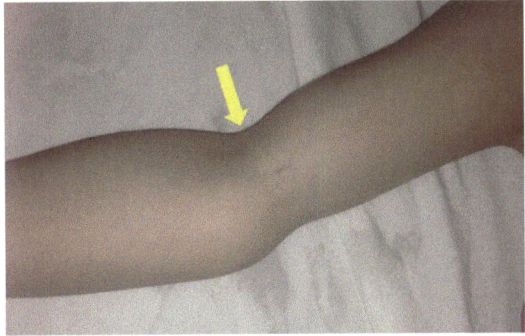

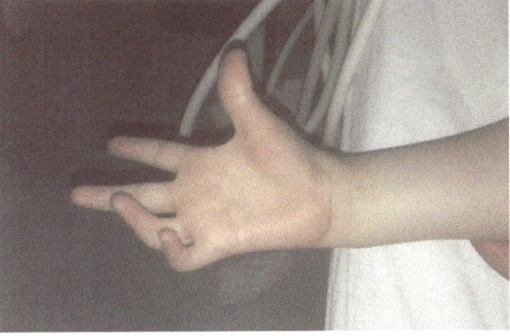

Fig. 4.93 External view of ulnar nerve absence. Note: the yellow arrow in the upper figure is pointing to the narrowing of the upper arm; the lower figure shows that the little finger is unable to stretch to a straight position

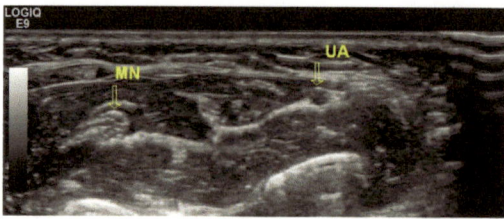

Fig. 4.94 Ultrasonogram of ulnar nerve absence. Note: *MN* short axis of the median nerve, *UA* ulnar artery

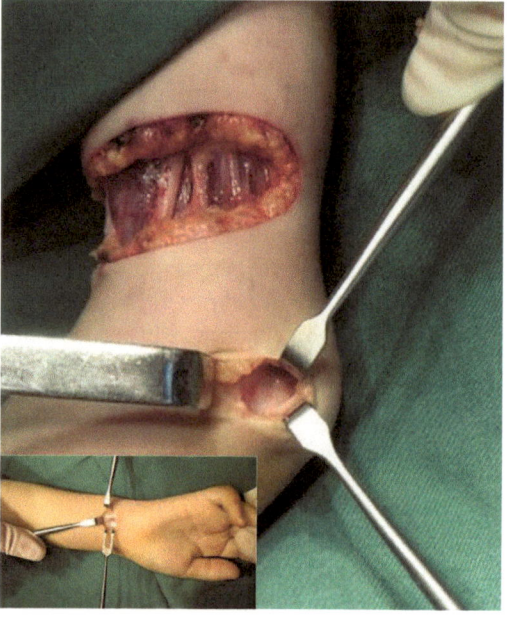

Fig. 4.95 Image of the operation for ulnar nerve absence

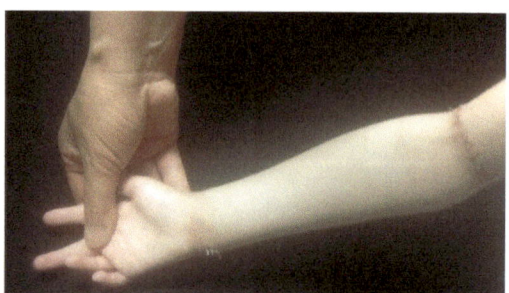

Fig. 4.96 External view after surgery for ulnar nerve absence

the indicators in ultrasonograms of cysts inside and outside a nerve and schwannoma, thereby offering a strong basis for clinical diagnosis and surgery. According to the position, cysts growing inside the epineurium are clinically termed intraneural cysts,

whereas those growing outside the endoneurium are termed extraneural cysts.

Case 37
See (Figs. 4.97 and 4.98) (Video 4.34).

ER 4.34 Dynamic image and explanation of ulnar nerve compression (formation of an extraneural cyst) in cubital tunnel syndrome

Case 38
See (Figs. 4.99, 4.100 and 4.101) (Video 4.35).

ER 4.35 Dynamic image and explanation of ulnar nerve compression (formation of an extraneural cyst) in cubital tunnel syndrome

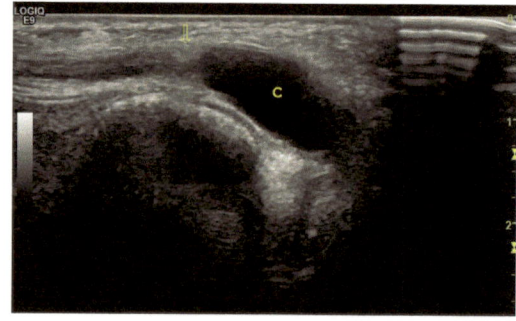

Fig. 4.97 Ultrasonogram of ulnar nerve entrapment (formation of an extraneural cyst) in cubital tunnel syndrome. Note: the arrow is pointing to the ulnar nerve, and C is an extraneural cyst of the ulnar nerve

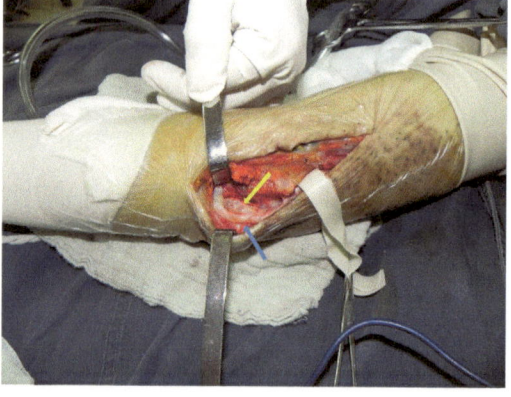

Fig. 4.98 Image of the operation for ulnar nerve entrapment (formation of an extraneural cyst) in cubital tunnel syndrome. Note: the blue arrow is pointing to the ulnar nerve and the yellow arrow is pointing to the extraneural cyst

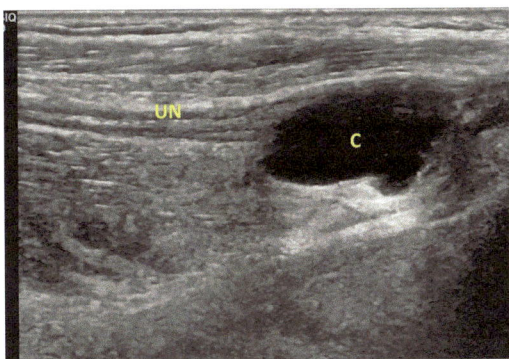

Fig. 4.99 Ultrasonogram of ulnar nerve entrapment (formation of an extraneural cyst) in cubital tunnel syndrome. Note: UN is the ulnar nerve and C is the extraneural cyst of the ulnar nerve

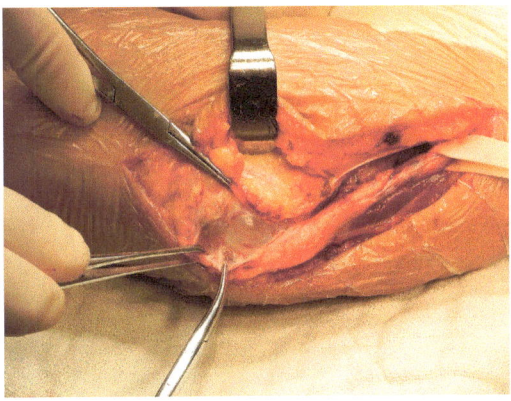

Fig. 4.100 Picture of the operation for ulnar nerve entrapment (formation of extraneural cyst) of cubital tunnel syndrome (before decollement)

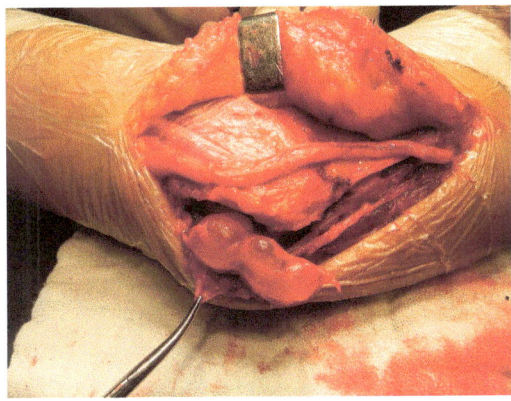

Fig. 4.101 Image of the operation for ulnar nerve entrapment (formation of an extraneural cyst) in cubital tunnel syndrome (after decollement)

Case 39

See (Figs. 4.102 and 4.103) (Video 4.36).

ER 4.36 Dynamic image and explanation of the formation of an intraneural cyst in the ulnar nerve in cubital tunnel syndrome

Case 40

See (Figs. 4.104 and 4.105) (Video 4.37).

ER 4.37 Dynamic image and explanation of the formation of an ulnar nerve extraneural cyst in cubital tunnel syndrome

Case 41

See (Figs. 4.106, 4.107 and 4.108).

Case 42

See (Figs. 4.109, 4.110 and 4.111) (Video 4.38).

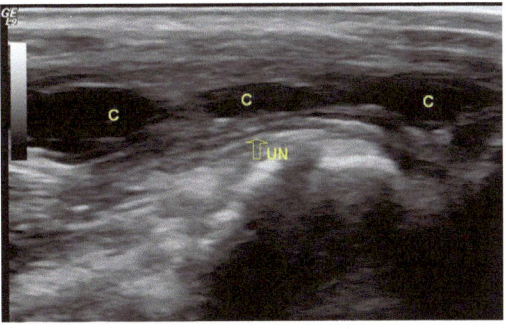

Fig. 4.102 Ultrasonogram of the formation of an ulnar nerve intraneural cyst in cubital tunnel syndrome. Note: UN is the ulnar nerve and C is the formation of an intraneural cyst in the ulnar nerve

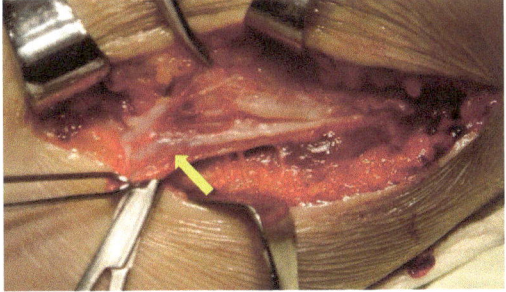

Fig. 4.103 Image of the operation for the formation of an ulnar nerve intraneural cyst in cubital tunnel syndrome. Note: the yellow arrow is pointing to the intraneural cyst of the ulnar nerve

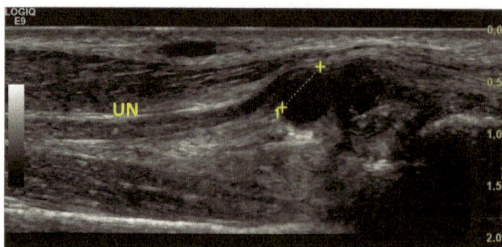

Fig. 4.104 Ultrasonogram of the formation of an ulnar nerve extraneural cyst in cubital tunnel syndrome. Note: UN is the ulnar nerve and the Vernier calliper shows the formation of an extraneural cyst of the ulnar nerve

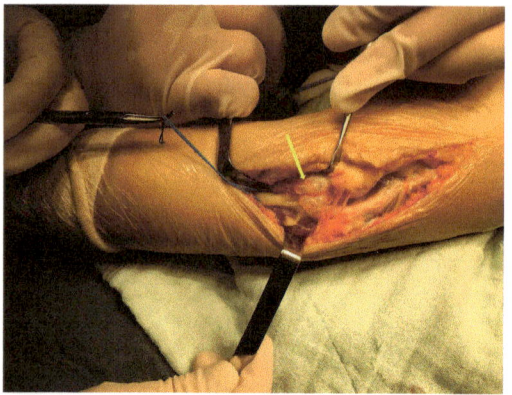

Fig. 4.105 Image of the operation for the formation of an ulnar nerve extraneural cyst in cubital tunnel syndrome. Note: the yellow arrow is pointing to the formation of an extraneural cyst of the ulnar nerve

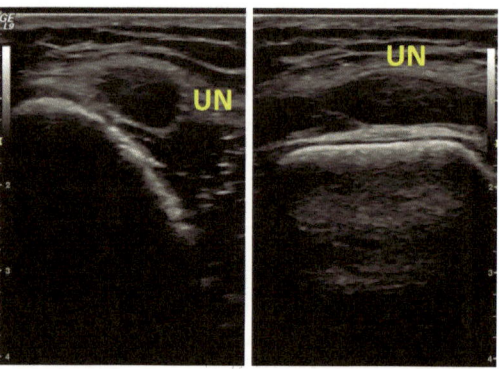

Fig. 4.106 Ultrasonogram of the formation of an ulnar nerve extraneural cyst in cubital tunnel syndrome. Note: UN indicates the wrapping of an extraneural cyst of the ulnar nerve

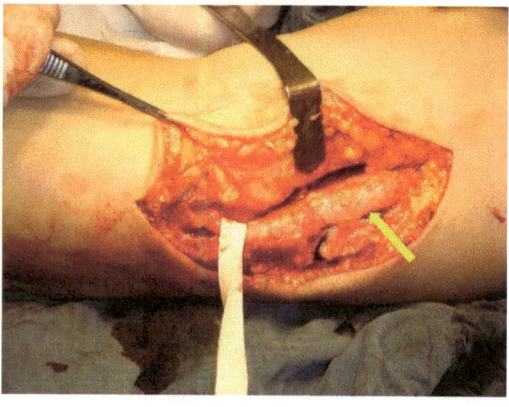

Fig. 4.107 Image of the operation for the formation of an ulnar nerve extraneural cyst in cubital tunnel syndrome (before decollement). Note: the yellow arrow is pointing to the wrapping of the extraneural cyst of the ulnar nerve before decollement

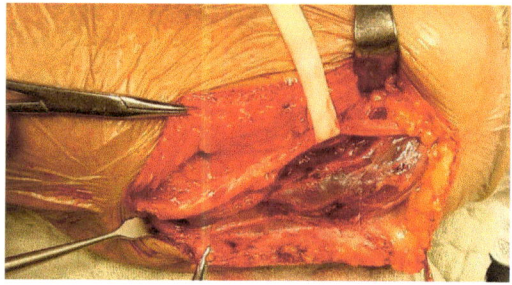

Fig. 4.108 Image of the operation for the formation of an ulnar nerve extraneural cyst in cubital tunnel syndrome (after decollement)

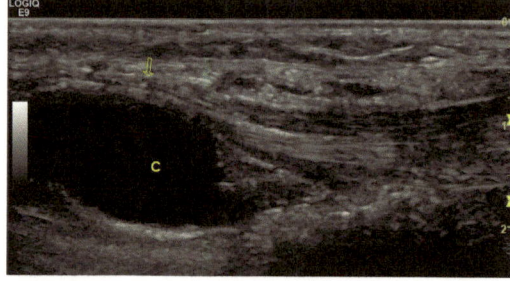

Fig. 4.109 Ultrasonogram of a superficial branch injury (formation of a cyst) of the ulnar nerve. Note: the arrow is pointing to the superficial branch of the ulnar nerve, and C is the cyst

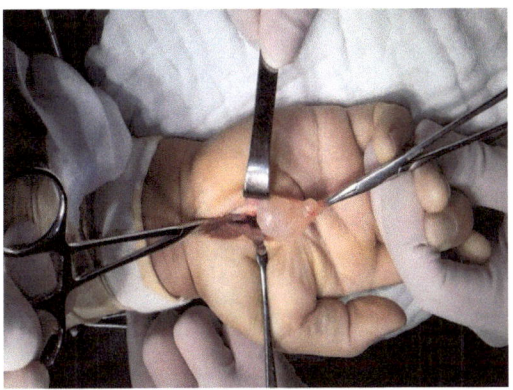

Fig. 4.110 Image of the operation for a superficial branch injury (formation of a cyst) of the ulnar nerve (before decollement)

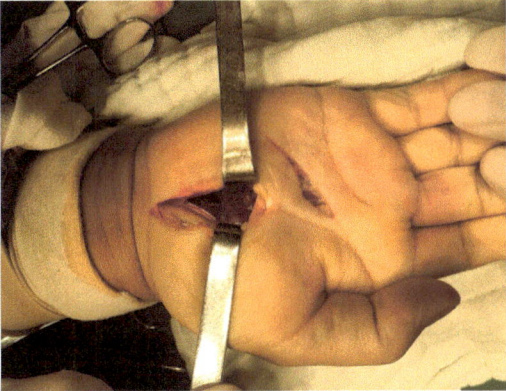

Fig. 4.111 Image of the operation for a superficial branch injury (formation of a cyst) of the ulnar nerve (after decollement)

ER 4.38 Dynamic image and explanation of a superficial branch injury (formation of a cyst) in the ulnar nerve

Summary Extraneural and intraneural cysts are a common cause of cubital tunnel syndrome. It is important to identify if the injury is caused by an extraneural cyst or an intraneural cyst for early diagnosis and treatment.

Notes 1. Peripheral extraneural cysts only compress the epineurium and cause little harm

to neural bundle branches; 2. Intraneural cysts are confined to the epineurium, and cyst fluid can directly compress and cause adhesion to neural bundle branches, thereby causing severe harm.

4.2.5 Radial Nerve (Including Interosseous Dorsal Nerve) Injury (Cases 43–52)

Quite a few patients suffer from peripheral nerve injury of unknown causes, and if they have mild or nontypical symptoms, the sonographer may not consider peripheral nerve injury in the initial examination. Therefore, awareness of such a disease must be raised [10]. Radial nerve paralysis caused by pulling and compressing the radial nerve and its branches for various reasons, and neural bundle torsion or constriction due to entrapment by repeated rotation of the forearm muscles are commonly seen in the upper limbs. The typical symptoms of such patients include unexplained weak extension of the wrists and fingers after upper limb movements, pain in the lateral and posterior upper arms or partial forearm, difficulty in retrieving objects, and even the occurrence of wrist drop. The clinical diagnosis of neural lesions of unknown causes in the upper limbs was traditionally based on judgement of the degree of neural injury by clinical performance and electrophysiological examination, but such a diagnosis is difficult to make because it is difficult to definitely determine the location and morphological changes of these neural lesions. High-frequency ultrasound can either clearly show the path and inner structure of the upper-limb radial nerve bundles or it can display the range covered by the constricted nerve bundles [11]. The ultrasonogram of the lesion shows constriction of part of the nerve, an enlarged hypoechoic nerve bundle at both ends, and the disappearance of an internal striped peri-neurium. In some cases, lesions are located in the interosseous dorsal nerve in the forearm, which is the deep branch of the radial nerve. In this case, the ultrasonogram shows that the nerve runs unevenly, that part of the nerve is thin and that the nerve bundle is enlarged at both ends, with an inner hypoechoic and hyperechoic epineurium.

Case 43

A female patient aged 16 years. This patient first had a cold and fever, and then suffered pains in the left lateral and posterior upper arm along with weak extension of wrists and fingers, and wrist drop for 2 months.

Electromyogram: Electrophysiological performance of upper-arm radial nerve injury.

Ultrasound finding: from the scanning on radial nerve, the nerve ran smoothly but was partially narrowed (2 mm in diameter) 1/3 of the way under the upper arm; the other part of the nerve was enlarged on both sides and presented tumour-like changes; the nerve was 1.0 cm in length, 0.35 cm in thickness and 0.16 cm² in cross-sectional area. Ultrasonic diagnosis: radial nerve injury (entrapment) on left upper arm with neuroma formation (Figs. 4.112 and 4.113) (Video 4.39).

Operation: the radial nerve of the left upper arm ran continuously and was partially narrowed 1/3 of the way under the upper arm; the nerve was also partly enlarged at both ends and featured degeneration and stripe-shaped tumour-like changes. Postoperative diagnosis: radial nerve injury of the left upper arm.

ER 4.39 Dynamic image and explanation of constriction of the radial nerve in the upper arm

Case 44

A female patient aged 17 years. Main complaint: the patient had left wrist drop for 1 month. Current medical history: the patient experienced weak extension of the left wrist and fingers, and pain and numbness of her left forearm. However, after

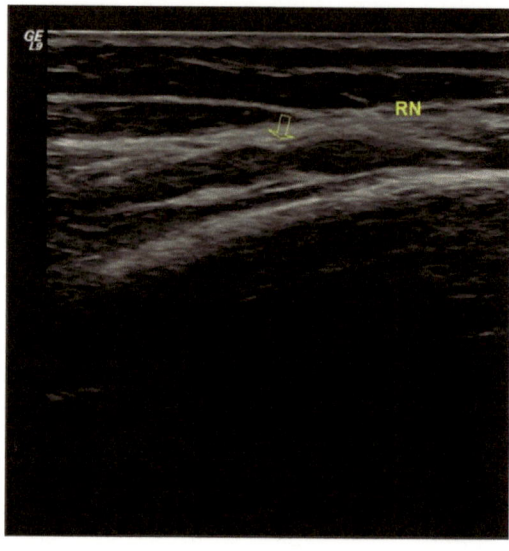

Fig. 4.112 Ultrasonogram of the constriction of the upper-arm radial nerve. Note: RN is the radial nerve and the arrow is pointing to constriction of the radial nerve

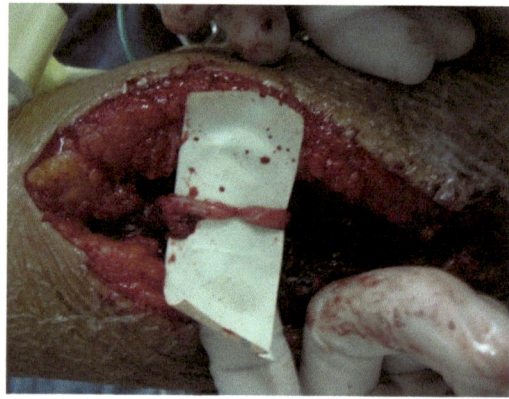

Fig. 4.113 Image of the operation for constriction of the upper-arm radial nerve

transfusion treatment (no details in medication) at a local hospital, the symptoms persisted and have recently deteriorated. Specialized physical examination: active extension restriction of the left wrist and related fingers, II-level force of the radial and ulnar wrist extensor muscles, numbness from the distal end of the left wrist crease and normal blood supply at the distal end of the fingers. Ultrasound finding: the left radial nerve, which ran smoothly and partly narrowed in the medial upper arm, had a diameter of 0.26 cm and a distal end diameter of 0.47 cm. Ultrasound diagnosis: the left radial nerve ran smoothly and partly narrowed inside the upper part of the upper arm, and thus partial constriction of the radial nerve was considered (Figs. 4.114, 4.115 and 4.116) (Video 4.40).

Operation: the radial nerve was obviously narrowed at 4 cm under the outlet of the radial nerve groove, with both ends connected only to the membrane; the lesion was 1.5 cm in length, with a hard texture and bead-shaped changes when touched; after removing the diseased neural tissue, the epineurium of the distal and proximal ends of the radial nerve was anastomosed.

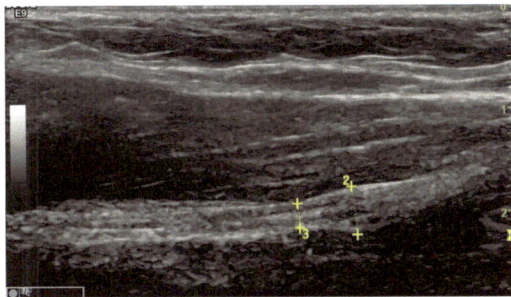

Fig. 4.114 Ultrasonogram of a radial nerve injury in the upper arm (sausage-shaped changes). Note: Vernier calliper 3 shows constriction of the radial nerve, and Vernier calliper 2 shows an enlarged radial nerve

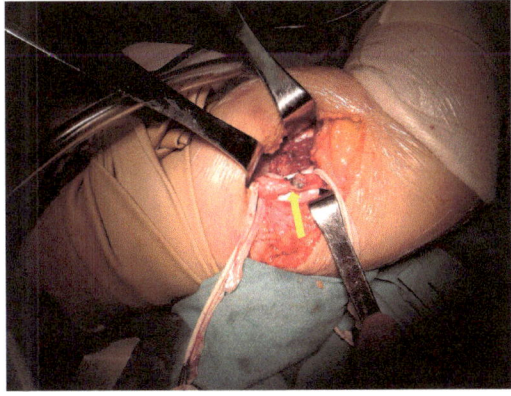

Fig. 4.115 Image of the operation for radial nerve injury of the upper arm (before repair). Note: the yellow arrow is pointing to constriction of the radial nerve

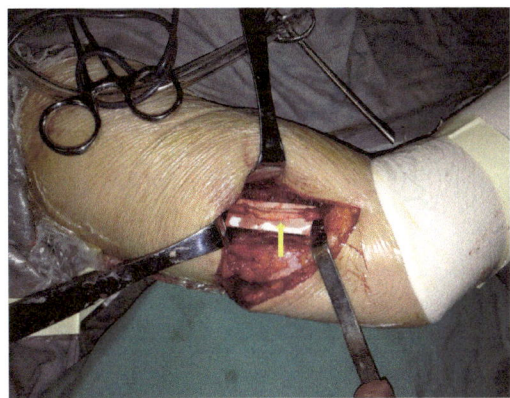

Fig. 4.116 Image of the operation for radial nerve injury of the upper arm (after repair). Note: the yellow arrow is pointing to the repaired radial nerve

ER 4.40 Dynamic image and explanation of radial nerve injury (sausage-shaped changes) in the upper arms

Case 45
See (Figs. 4.117 and 4.118).

Case 46
See (Figs. 4.119 and 4.120) (Video 4.41).

ER 4.41 Dynamic image and explanation of the vasculature running across the dorsal interosseous nerve

Case 47
A male patient aged 45 years. Main complaint: functional restriction of the active extension of all the fingers of the right hand for over 9 months. Current medical history: the patient experienced functional obstacles of active extension of all the fingers of the right hand with no obvious cause 9 months earlier. Specialized physical examination: abnormities of finger drop were observed on his right hand, while his dorsal right hand was swollen. All the fingers of his right hand were unable to extend, with 0-level muscle force of the extensor longus pollicis and extensor digitorum and ability for passive movements. Pressing pain occurred at 1/3 of the middle and upper parts of the right dorsal forearm. Electromyogram: the injury was likely interosseous dorsal nerve injury of the right forearm.

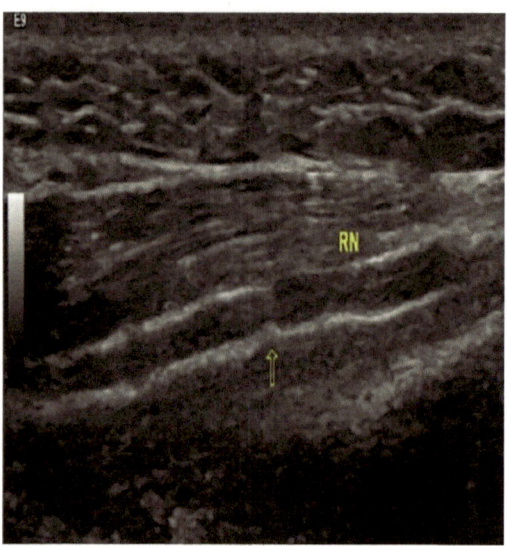

Fig. 4.117 Ultrasonogram of multiple constrictions of the radial nerve in the upper arm. Note: RN is the radial nerve, and the arrow is pointing to constriction of the radial nerve

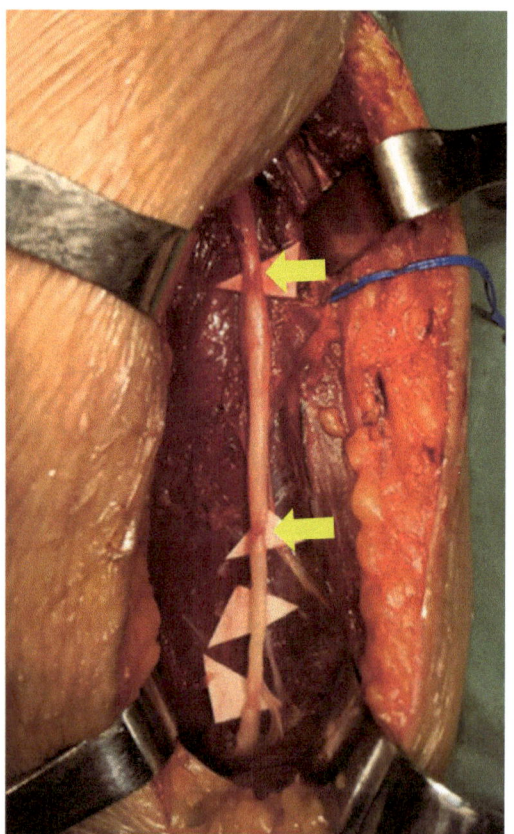

Fig. 4.118 Image of the operation for multiple constrictions of the radial nerve in the upper arm. Note: the yellow arrow is pointing to multiple constrictions of the radial nerve

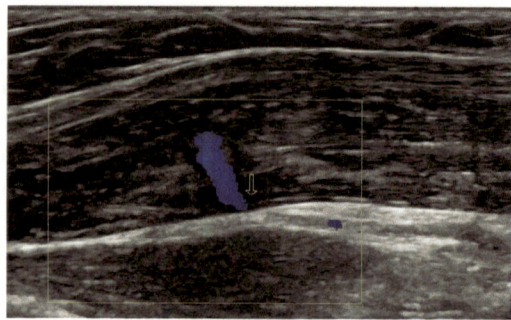

Fig. 4.119 Colour Doppler ultrasonogram of the vasculature running across the dorsal interosseous nerve. Note: the arrow is pointing to the vasculature running across the dorsal interosseous nerve

Ultrasonic finding: the interosseous dorsal nerve in the upper part of the right forearm was uneven, with a slightly hypoechoic area; the nerve was 1.2 mm in diameter at its thinner part and 1.5 mm at its wider part. Ultrasound diagnosis: the interosseous dorsal nerve in the upper part of the right forearm was uneven, and neural inflammatory changes were not excluded (Figs. 4.121 and 4.122) (Video 4.42).

Operation: during surgery, it was found that the deep branch of the radial nerve became thin at the arch of the supinator tendon and that part of the deep branch of the radial nerve became flat and thin after incision of the supinator on the deep branch surface of the radial nerve. The nerve was then completely loosened.

ER 4.42 Dynamic image and explanation of interosseous dorsal nerve injury

Case 48
See (Figs. 4.123 and 4.124).

Case 49
See (Figs. 4.125, 4.126 and 4.127) (Video 4.43).

ER 4.43 Dynamic image and explanation of multiple constrictions of the radial nerve in the upper arm

Case 50
See (Fig. 4.128).

Case 51
See (Figs. 4.129 and 4.130) (Video 4.44).

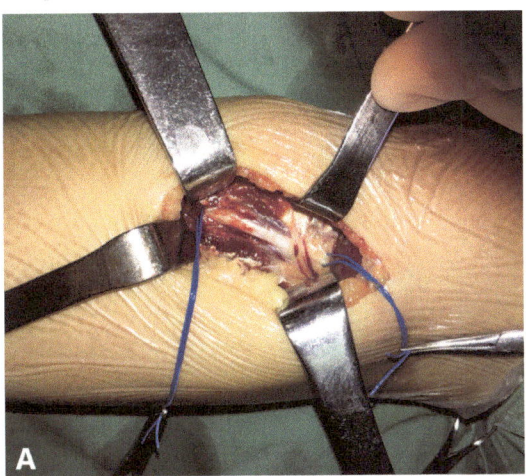
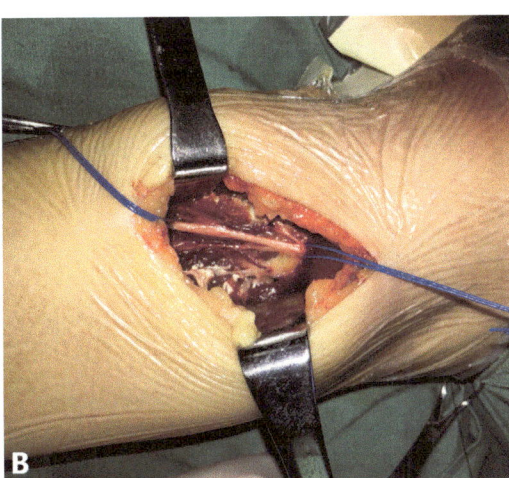

Fig. 4.120 Image of the vasculature running across the dorsal interosseous nerve during surgery. Note: (**a**): the vasculature running across the dorsal interosseous nerve (arrows), (**b**): released interosseous dorsal nerve after riding blood vessels occlusion

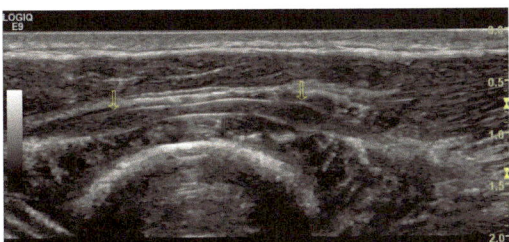

Fig. 4.121 Ultrasonogram of an interosseous dorsal nerve injury. Note: the arrow is pointing to the interosseous dorsal nerve injury

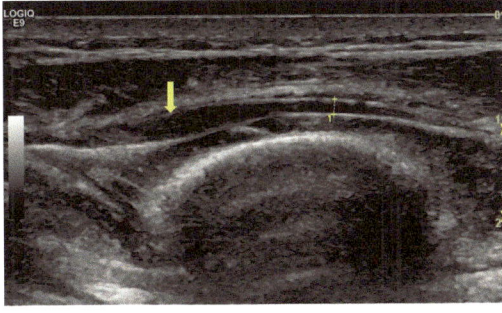

Fig. 4.123 Ultrasonogram of an interosseous dorsal nerve injury. Note: Vernier calliper indicates the interosseous dorsal nerve and the yellow arrow is pointing to the partially enlarged interosseous dorsal nerve

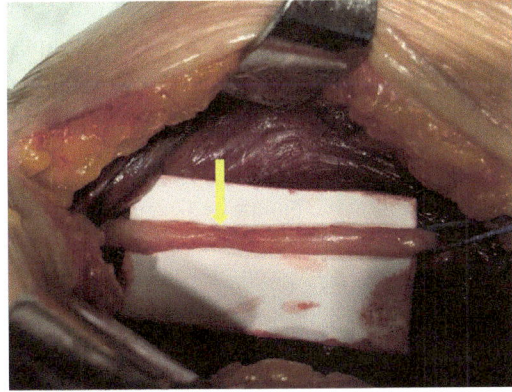

Fig. 4.122 Image of the operation for interosseous dorsal nerve injury. Note: the yellow arrow is pointing to the narrowing of the interosseous dorsal nerve

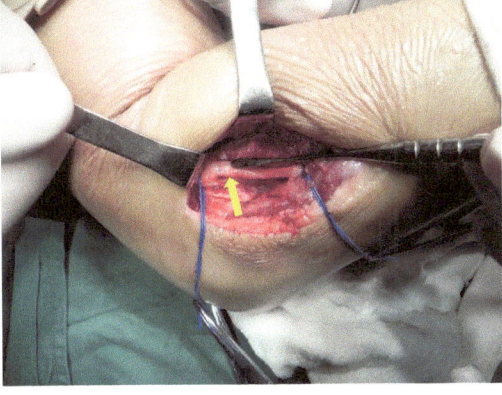

Fig. 4.124 Image of the operation for interosseous dorsal nerve injury. Note: the yellow arrow is pointing to the partially enlarged interosseous dorsal nerve

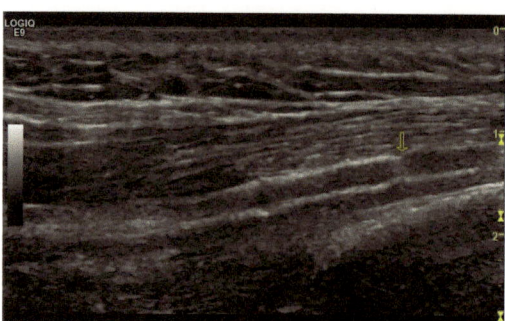

Fig. 4.125 Ultrasonogram of multiple constrictions of the radial nerve in the upper arm. Note: the yellow arrow is pointing to constrictions of the radial nerve

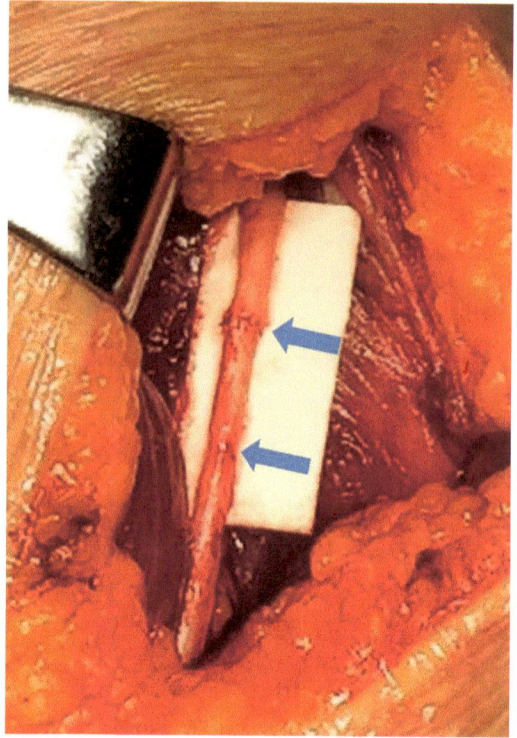

Fig. 4.127 Image of the operation for multiple constrictions of the radial nerve in the upper arm (after repair). Note: the blue arrow is pointing to the repaired radial nerve

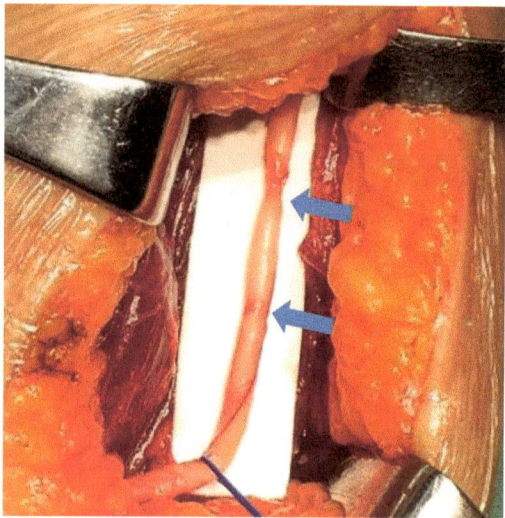

Fig. 4.126 Image of the operation for multiple constrictions of the radial nerve in the upper arm (before repair). Note: the blue arrow is pointing to multiple constrictions of the radial nerve

ER 4.44 Dynamic image and explanation of a radial nerve fracture in the upper arm

Case 52
See (Figs. 4.131 and 4.132).

Summary Viral infection may cause radial nerve inflammatory injury. First, the virus causes whole-body infection, fever, aches and pains, and then the viral infection causes deterioration of the lesion based on previous anatomy (such as partial compression caused by the lateral head of the triceps brachii muscle), thereby generating the symptoms of radial nerve injury in the upper arms. These injuries can also be caused by improper force on and use of the upper arm or poor body position (e.g., long-term compression of the upper arm during sleep after alcohol-induced impairment). The repeated movements after injury will further affect the nerve, thus causing fibrosis and self-constriction of the radial nerve bundle and even vasculitis in severe cases [12].

Notes 1. Weakness of the upper limbs, inability to grab objects and even wrist drop in serious cases are the most common clinical features of radial nerve injury in the upper arms; 2. Interosseous dorsal nerve injury often shows obvious pressing pain in the forearms; 3. During ultrasonic examination, attention should be paid to the continuity of

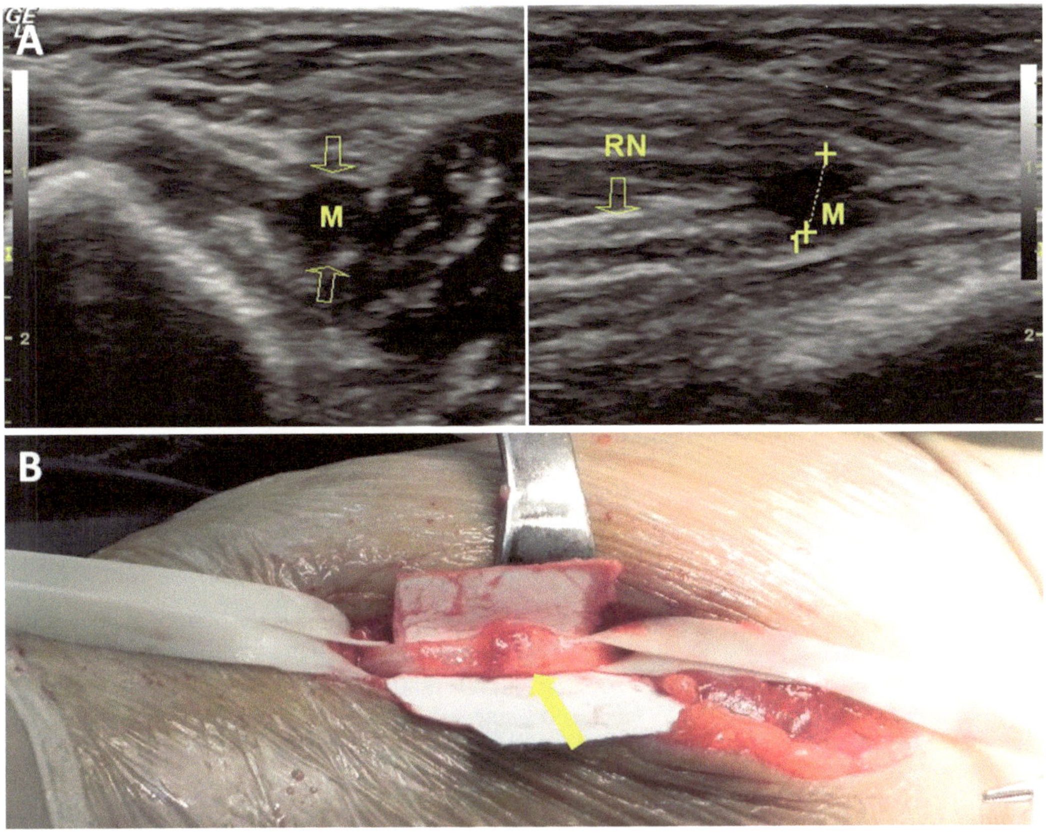

Fig. 4.128 Ultrasonogram and surgical image of a traumatic neuroma of the radial nerve in the upper arm. Note: in (**a**), RN is the radial nerve, and M is the short and long axes of a traumatic neuroma; in (**b**), the yellow arrow is pointing to the traumatic neuroma of the radial nerve

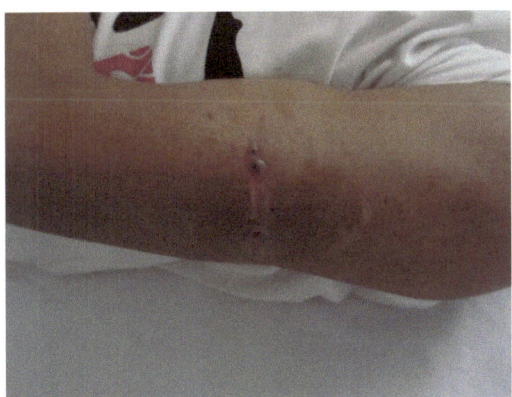

Fig. 4.129 External view of a radial nerve fracture in the upper arm

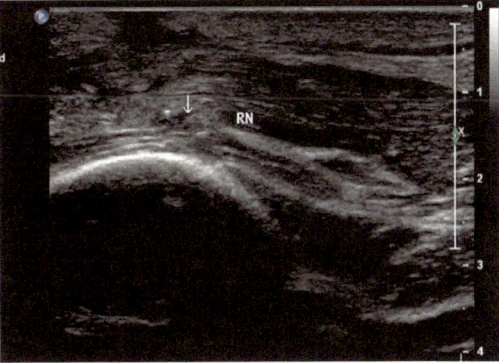

Fig. 4.130 Ultrasonogram of a radial nerve fracture in the upper arm. Note: RN is the radial nerve, and the arrow is pointing to the radial nerve fracture

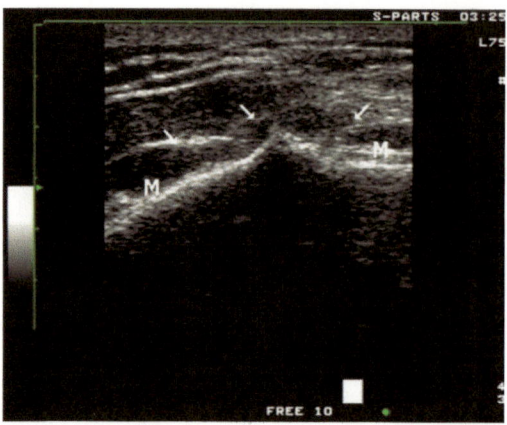

Fig. 4.131 Ultrasonogram of a radial nerve fracture in the upper arm. Note: the arrow is pointing to the radial nerve fracture, and M is the formation of a traumatic neuroma due to radial nerve fracture

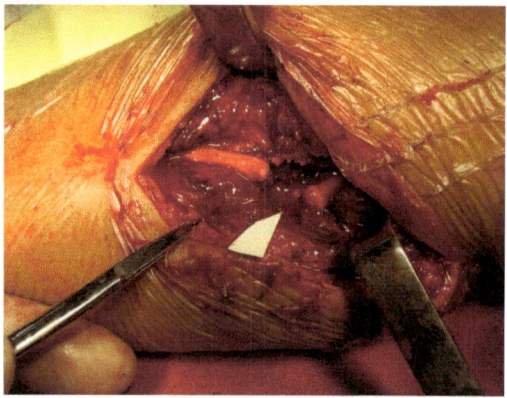

Fig. 4.132 Image of the operation for radial nerve fracture in the upper arm

the interosseous dorsal nerve and radial nerve in the upper arms to determine whether the nerve has constriction, fracture, enlargement or oedema, thereby correctly judging the injury position.

4.2.6 Peripheral Schwannoma in the Upper Limbs (Cases 53–61)

Both schwannoma and neurofibroma are termed nerve sheath tumours, which often grow on greater nerve trunks under the skin and in the superficial muscular layer. Therefore, inexperienced sonographers often diagnose such tumours as haematomas, thrombi or haemangiomas. Their ultrasound features include hypoechoic mass, clear boundaries, an external membrane and enhanced echo at the rear. Pathologically, schwannomas have an external membrane. During surgical resection, it is easy to completely remove the tumour without harming the nerve trunk.

Case 53

A male patient aged 66 years. Main complaint: a mass on the left wrist along with numbness of the left hand for 7 months. Current medical history: the patient found a raised, hard mass on his left wrist with no obvious cause 7 months ago, with pressing pains radiating to the forearm. Specialized physical examination: a hard-textured mass 1 × 2 cm in size was found on the left wrist; the mass had a blurred boundary with surrounding tissues and obvious burn, pressing pain that radiated to the second to fourth fingers. The interosseous muscle of the left hand was obviously atrophied; the patient also experienced weakness when opening and closing the fingers; movement of the thumb towards the palm was confined, and the patient experienced obvious numbness of the second to fourth fingers, and the radial artery pulse could be felt.

Ultrasound finding: along the path of the median nerve at the left wrist was a mixed echo zone of 2.8 cm × 1.7 cm, with a clear boundary, regular form and connection to the nerve. CDFI showed the scattered and bar-shaped blood flow signals in the solid portion. Ultrasound diagnosis: the mixed mass in the path of the median nerve at the left wrist was considered a schwannoma (Figs. 4.133 and 4.134) (Video 4.45).

Operation: during surgery, the median nerve at the left wrist presented fusiform changes, and the round mass compressed the nerve bundle branch. It was found that the bundle branch was complete and that it connected with fewer skin branches after the outer membrane was incised to completely separate the mass from the nerve bundle. The median nerve was loosened towards the distal and proximal ends.

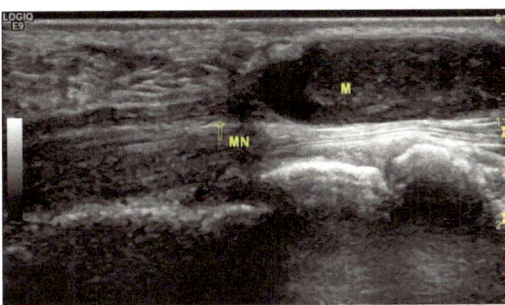

Fig. 4.133 Ultrasonogram of a schwannoma of the median nerve at the wrist. Note: MN is the median nerve, and M is the median nerve schwannoma

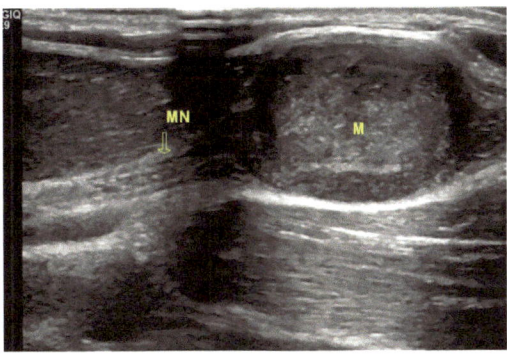

Fig. 4.135 Ultrasonogram of a schwannoma of the median nerve in the upper arm. Note: MN is the median nerve, and M is the median nerve schwannoma

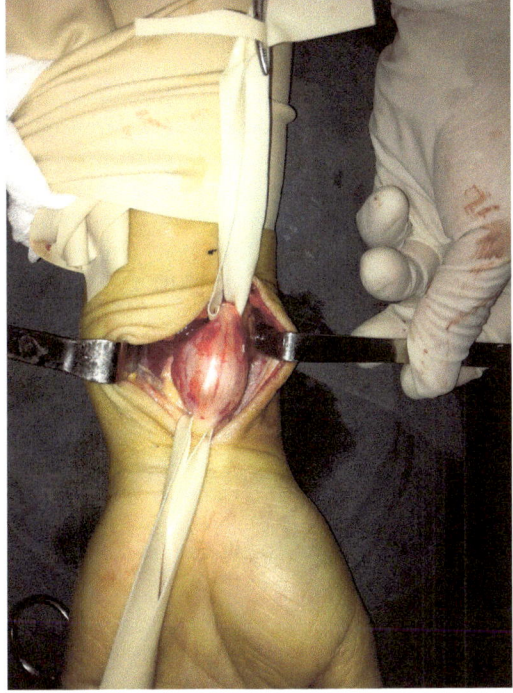

Fig. 4.134 Image of the operation for a median nerve schwannoma at the wrist

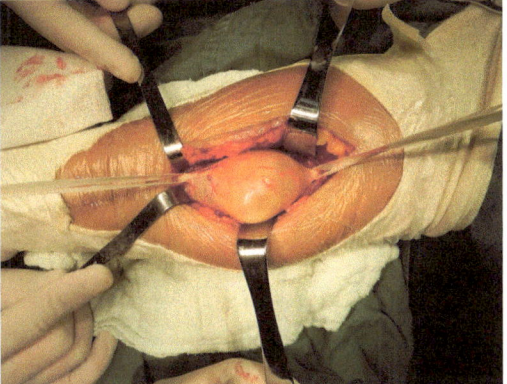

Fig. 4.136 Image of the operation for median nerve schwannoma in the upper arm

ER 4.46 Dynamic image and explanation of schwannoma of the median nerve in the upper arm

ER 4.47 Dynamic image and explanation of CEUS of a median nerve schwannoma in the upper arm

Pathology: cellular schwannoma with cystic changes at the left wrist and active hyperplasia indicative of a partial oncocytoma.

ER 4.45 Dynamic image and explanation of a schwannoma of the median nerve at the wrist

Case 54
See (Figs. 4.135 and 4.136) (Videos 4.46 and 4.47).

Case 55
A male patient aged 48 years. Main complaint: a mass in his left upper arm that persisted for 12 years and that started growing larger 1 year earlier. Current medical history: the patient found a painless soybean-sized mass on the inner side of the upper part of his left upper arm without an obvious cause 12 years ago, but the mass was not examined and treated at that time. One year ago,

the patient found that the mass began increasing in size, which was accompanied by numbness in the little finger with pressing pain; the numbness and pain deteriorated after hard work, and the symptoms were relieved after rest. Therefore, the patient presented to our hospital for ultrasonic examination, after which a hypoechoic zone approximately 2.0 cm × 1.5 cm in size was seen in the path of the ulnar nerve in the left upper arm, with a clear boundary and regular form. Ultrasound diagnosis: ulnar nerve schwannoma of the left upper arm (Figs. 4.137, 4.138, 4.139 and 4.140). Operation: after incision of the skin on the left upper arm, a hard tumour 2.0 × 3.0 cm in size with a clear boundary and homogenous density was found, and the membrane around it also surrounded the ulnar nerve bundle and small cutaneous nerves. After the tumour was com-

pletely removed, it was diagnosed as an ulnar nerve schwannoma.

Case 56
See (Figs. 4.141 and 4.142) (Video 4.48).

ER 4.48 Dynamic image and explanation of radial nerve schwannoma at the axilla

Case 57
See (Figs. 4.143 and 4.144) (Videos 4.49 and 4.50).

ER 4.49 Dynamic image and explanation of radial nerve schwannoma

ER 4.50 Explanation of radial nerve schwannoma during surgery

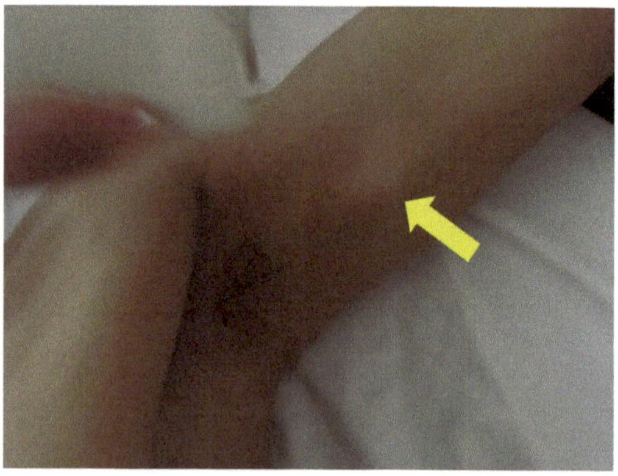

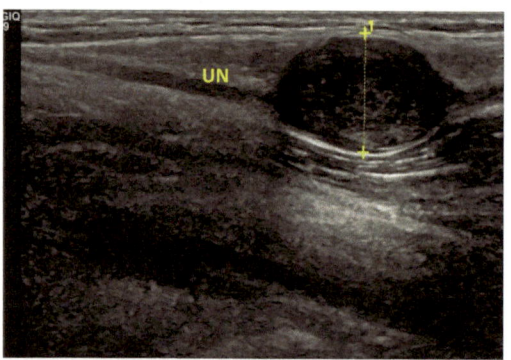

Fig. 4.137 External view of an ulnar nerve schwannoma in the upper arm. Note: the yellow arrow indicates the superficial mass

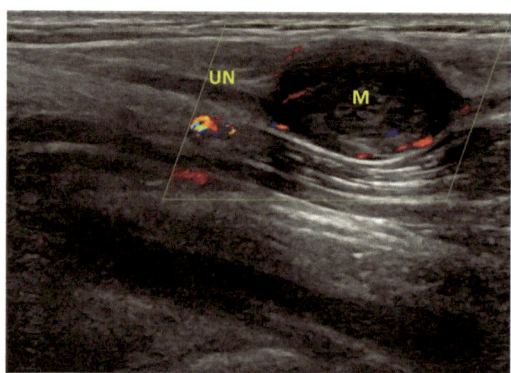

Fig. 4.139 Colour Doppler image of an ulnar nerve schwannoma in the upper arm. Note: UN is the ulnar nerve, and M is the ulnar nerve schwannoma

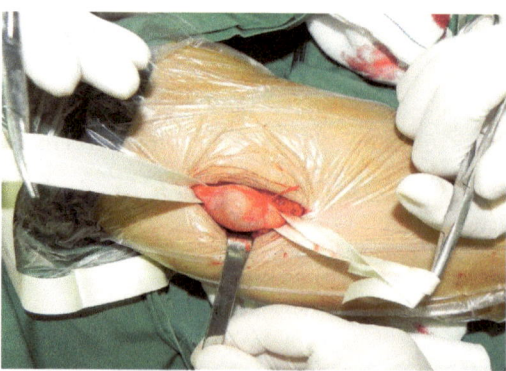

Fig. 4.138 2D ultrasonogram of ulnar nerve schwannoma in the upper arm. Note: UN is the ulnar nerve, and at the Vernier calliper is the ulnar nerve schwannoma

Fig. 4.140 Image of the operation for ulnar nerve schwannoma in the upper arm

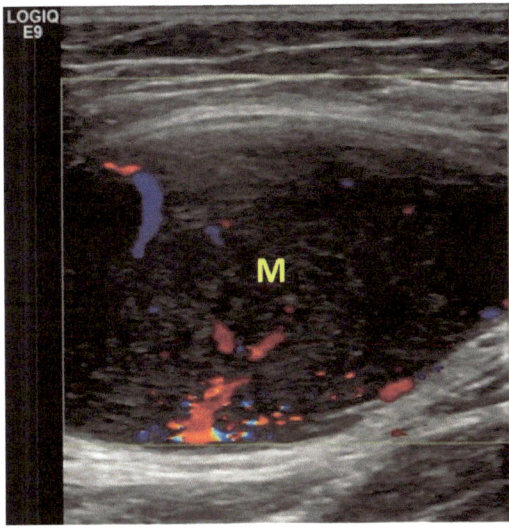

Fig. 4.141 Ultrasonogram of a radial nerve schwannoma at the axilla. Note: M is the radial nerve schwannoma

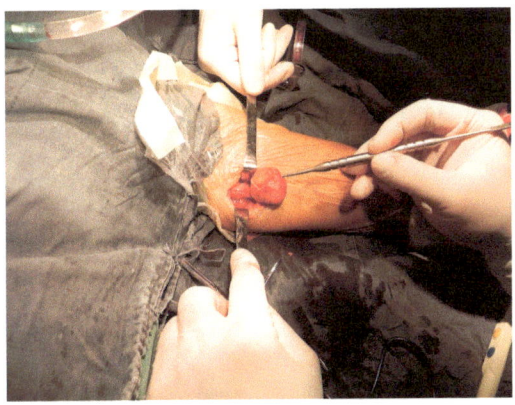

Fig. 4.142 Image of the operation for radial nerve schwannoma at the axilla

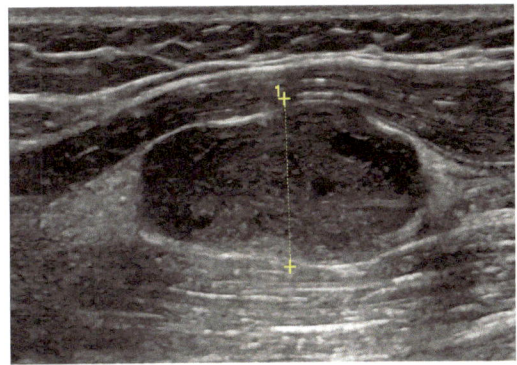

Fig. 4.143 Ultrasonogram of a radial nerve schwannoma. Note: The Vernier calliper indicates a radial nerve schwannoma

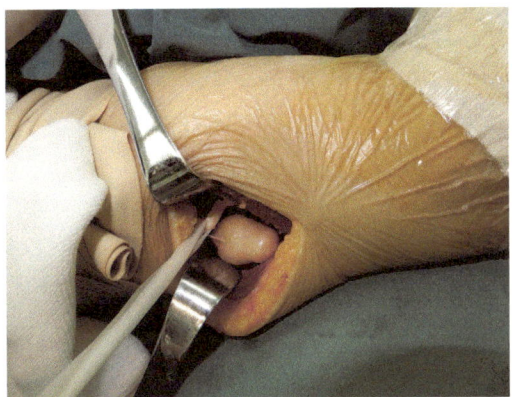

Fig. 4.144 Image of the operation for radial nerve schwannoma

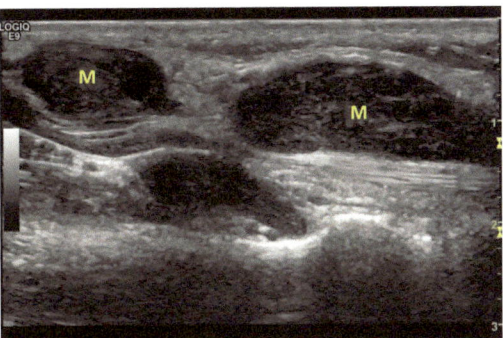

Fig. 4.145 Ultrasonogram of multiple schwannomas in the upper limb. Note: M indicates the schwannomas

Case 58
See (Figs. 4.145, 4.146 and 4.147) (Video 4.51).

ER 4.51 Dynamic image and explanation of multiple schwannomas in the upper limb

Case 59
See (Figs. 4.148 and 4.149) (Videos 4.52 and 4.53).

ER 4.52 Dynamic image and explanation of ulnar nerve schwannoma

ER 4.53 Explanation of ulnar nerve schwannoma during surgery

Case 60
See (Figs. 4.150, 4.151 and 4.152) (Videos 4.54 and 4.55).

ER 4.54 Dynamic image and explanation of multiple schwannomas

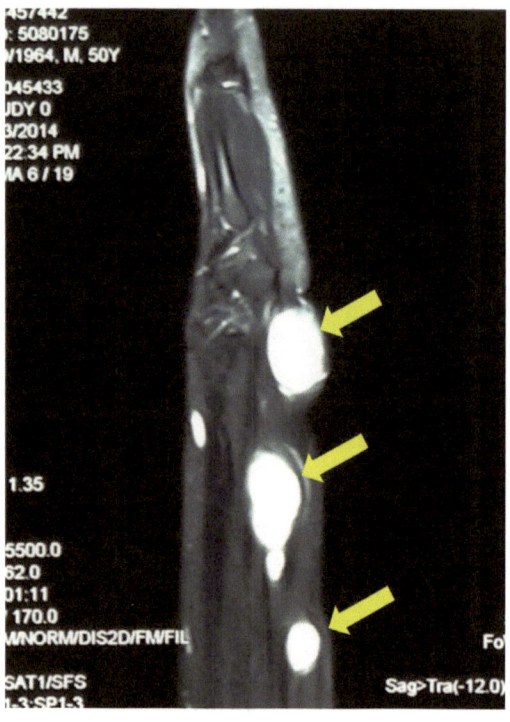

Fig. 4.146 MRI of multiple schwannomas in the upper limb. Note: the yellow arrows indicate the schwannomas

ER 4.55 Explanation of multiple schwannomas during surgery

Case 61

See (Figs. 4.153 and 4.154).

Summary In cases where a mass is found in the upper limbs, especially in the muscular layer, it

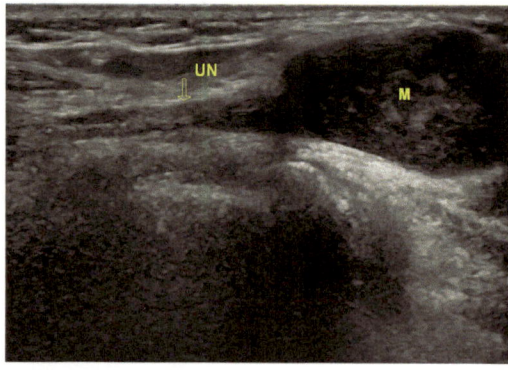

Fig. 4.148 Ultrasonogram of an ulnar nerve schwannoma. Note: the arrow indicates the ulnar nerve, and M is the ulnar nerve schwannoma

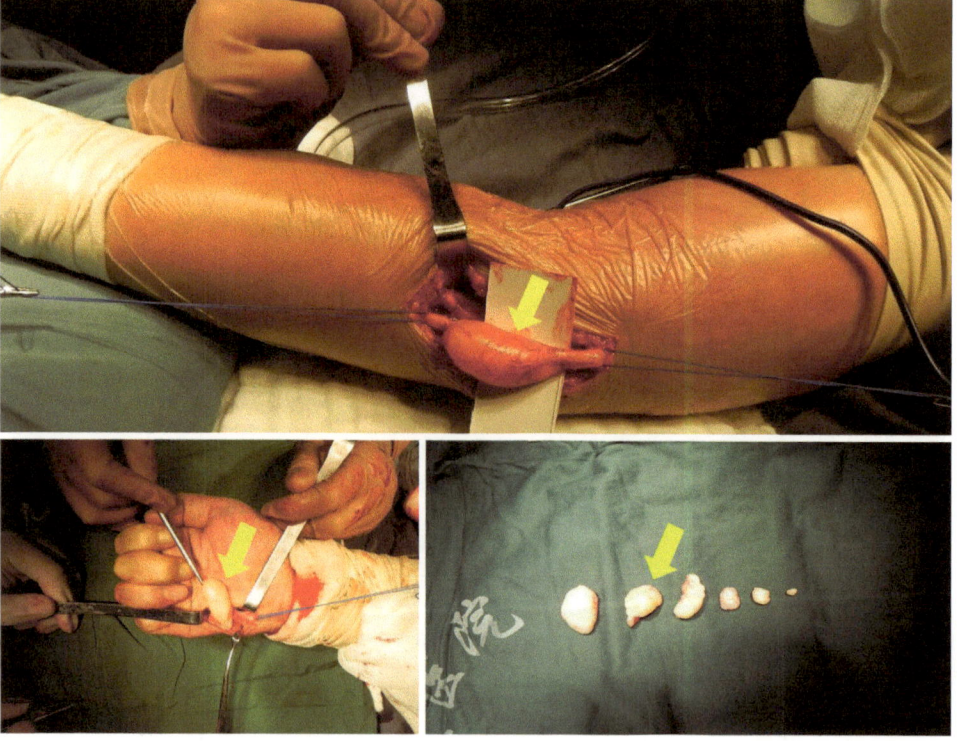

Fig. 4.147 Image of the operation for multiple schwannomas in the upper limb. Note: the yellow arrow indicates the schwannomas

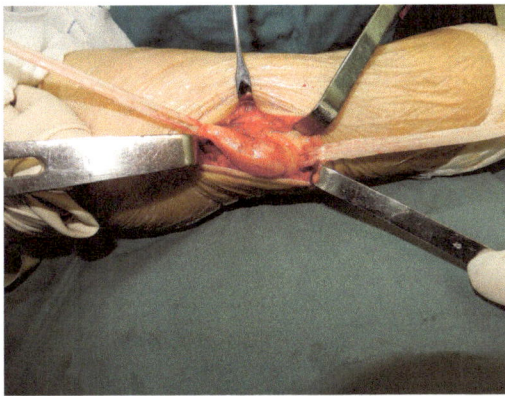

Fig. 4.149 Image of the operation for ulnar nerve schwannoma

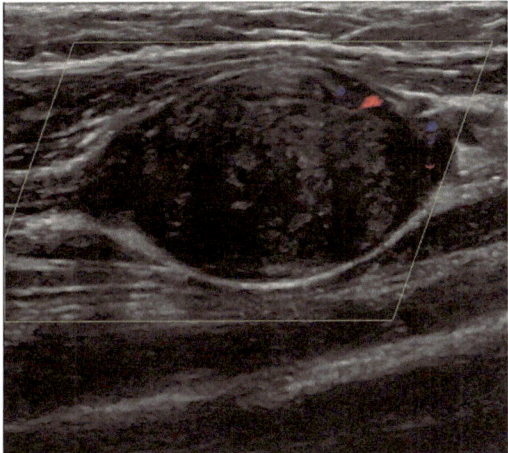

Fig. 4.150 Colour Doppler ultrasonogram of multiple schwannomas. Note: M is the median nerve schwannoma

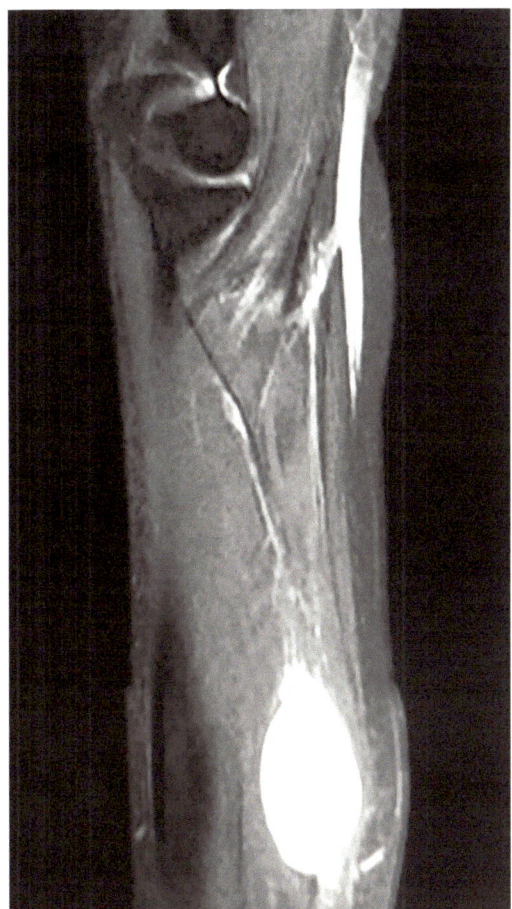

Fig. 4.151 MRI of multiple schwannomas. Note: the arrow indicates the schwannoma

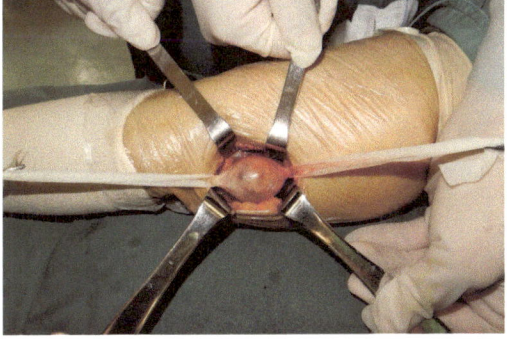

Fig. 4.152 Image of the operation for multiple schwannomas

should first be considered that the mass is derived from a nerve. The sonographer should be familiar with the anatomical routes of peripheral nerves and their neighbouring connections. During scanning, the connection of the mass with nerves should be observed, while identifying it as a lipoma, fascia nodule, haemangioma, enlarged lymph nodes or tendon. Ultrasonic examination is of great clinical value in diagnosing the causes of peripheral soft tissue masses, as it helps to find and confirm the relationship between a tumour and nerves and the formation of neuromas; ultrasound also offers plenty of information with regard to the combination of clinical symptoms and signs, which is useful for surgery.

Notes 1. Nerve sheath tumours often present as hypoechoic lumps, but other superficial soft tissue lumps may also be hypoechoic, and these can be identified by the anatomy of normal nerves and the features of the sonogram; 2. The connection of

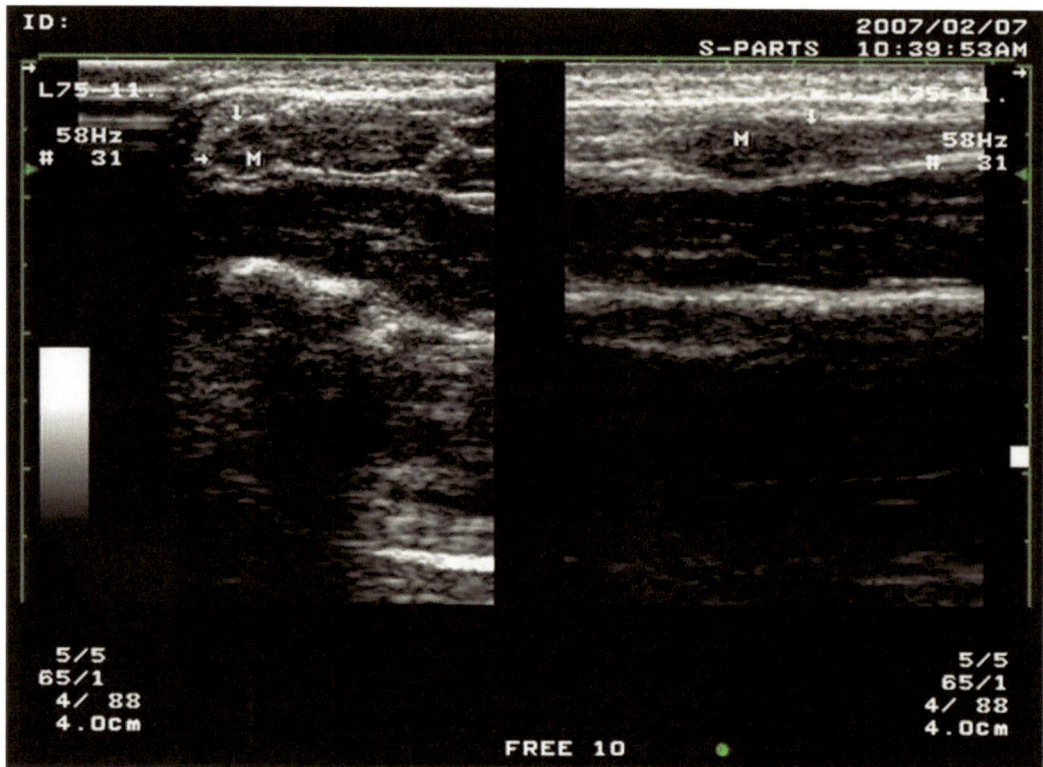

Fig. 4.153 Ultrasonogram of a schwannoma of the digital nerve. Note: the arrow indicates the digital nerve, and M is the digital nerve schwannoma

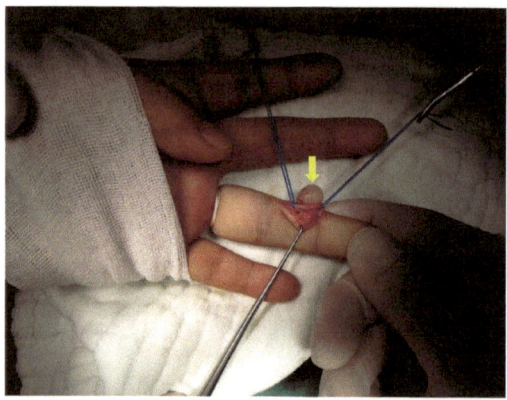

Fig. 4.154 Image of the operation for digital nerve schwannoma. Note: the yellow arrow indicates the digital nerve schwannoma

tumours to nerves is a major sign for locating a neurogenic tumour; 3. Pressing pain and numbness are also key points in the differentiation of these tumours from other non-neurogenic soft tissue lumps in the limbs.

4.2.7 Neurolipomatosis (Cases 62–63)

Neurolipomatosis, also known as neural fibrolipomatosis, is a type of rare and benign peripheral nerve lesion that often grows in the median nerve and is accompanied by macrodactylia of the affected limbs; the sonogram shows hypoechoic nerve fibres and hyperechoic fatty tissues that intertwine with each other, presenting a lotus root array with a thickened nerve tract.

Case 62
See (Figs. 4.155, 4.156 and 4.157) (Video 4.56).

ER 4.56 Dynamic image and explanation of ulnar nerve neurolipomatosis

Case 63
A male patient aged 39 years. Main complaint: the patient suffered amyotrophy of his right upper arm

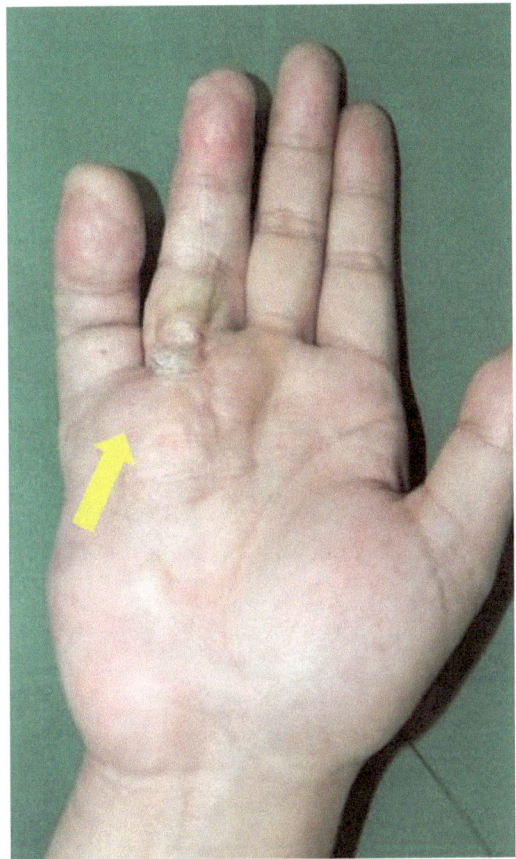

Fig. 4.155 External view of neurolipomatosis of the ulnar nerve. Note: the yellow arrow is pointing to the lesion

in the last 2 years, especially his deltoid and musculus biceps brachii, without obvious causes. Physical examination: the right upper arm showed amyotrophy below the shoulder and above the elbow. Ultrasound diagnosis: partial fatty infiltration of the musculocutaneous nerve (Figs. 4.158, 4.159, 4.160, 4.161 and 4.162) (Video 4.57). MRI finding: long T1 signals are found at the right axillary nerve root, and thus partial neural fatty infiltration and amyotrophy of the right upper arm were considered. Postoperative pathology: a hyperplastic fibrous texture, vascular tissue and adipose tissue were seen (beside the right brachial plexus).

ER 4.57 Dynamic image and explanation of nerve fibre fatty infiltration of the musculocutaneous nerve in the upper limb

Summary The two cases above suggested that, when patients experience symptoms such as visibly enlarged fingers and upper arm amyotrophy, diseases related to nerves should be considered first; the above lesions were located between the muscle and fat tissue layer, and thus inexperienced sonographers may diagnose such lesions as lipomyomas. Therefore, examiners should be familiar with the anatomical structure and the routes of the ulnar nerve and musculocutaneous nerve to make a correct diagnosis of neural lesions.

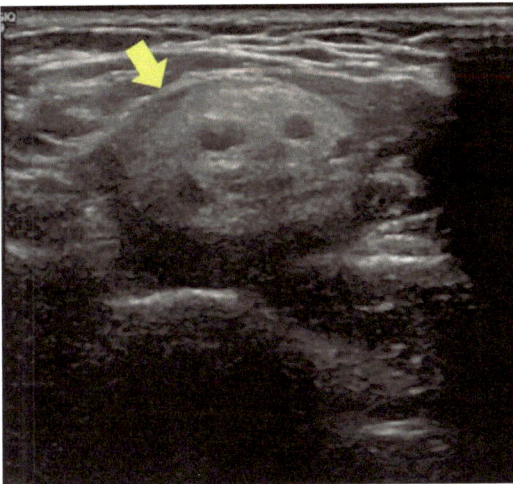
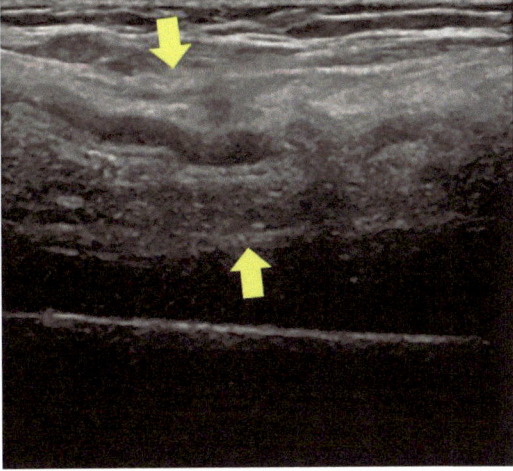

Fig. 4.156 Ultrasonogram of neurolipomatosis of the ulnar nerve. Note: the yellow arrow is pointing to the short and long axes of fibrous fatty infiltration of the ulnar nerve

Fig. 4.157 Image of
the operation for ulnar
nerve neurolipomatosis.
Note: the yellow arrow
is pointing to ulnar
nerve neurolipomatosis

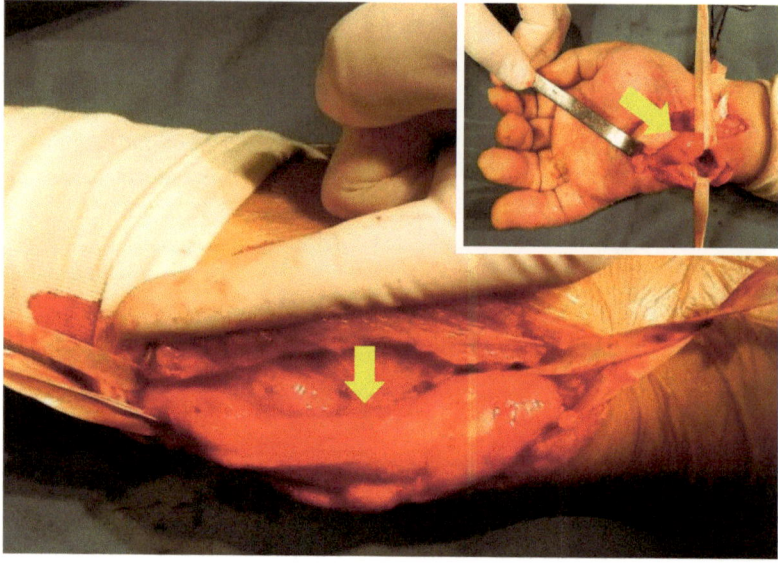

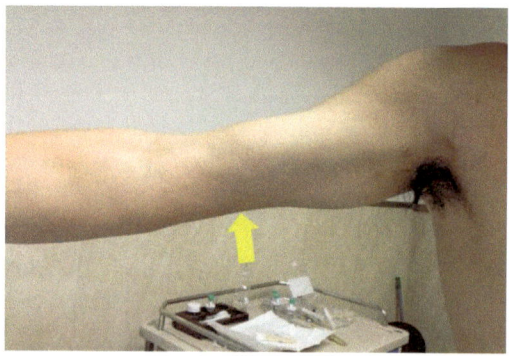

Fig. 4.158 External view of nerve fibre fatty infiltration
of the musculocutaneous nerve in the upper limb. Note:
the yellow arrow is pointing to amyotrophy of the upper
arm

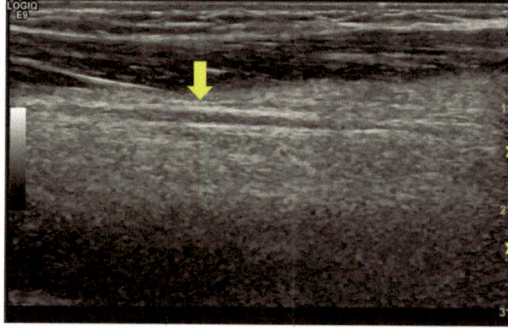

Fig. 4.160 Ultrasonogram of nerve fibre fatty infiltration
of the musculocutaneous nerve in the upper limb (longitudinal section). Note: the yellow arrow is pointing to the
long axis of the abnormal echo of nerve fibre fatty
infiltration

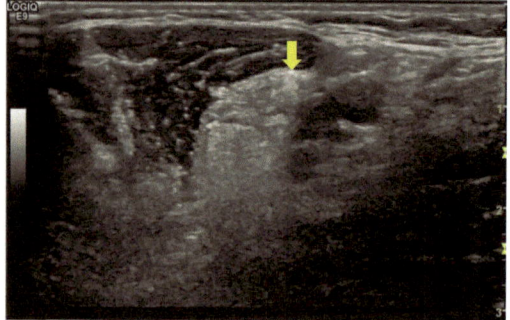

Fig. 4.159 Ultrasonogram of nerve fibre fatty infiltration
of the musculocutaneous nerve in the upper limb (cross
section). Note: the yellow arrow is pointing to the short
axis of the abnormal echo of nerve fibre fatty infiltration

4.3 Typical Cases of Neurological Diseases of the Lower Limbs

The nerves in the lower limbs mainly include
the sciatic nerve, tibial nerve, common peroneal nerve, femoral nerve and saphenous nerve.
High-frequency ultrasound can clearly show
their paths and fine structures and can also pinpoint their positions, ranges and relationships to
the surrounding tissues in cases of neural injuries
by comparative examination with the uninjured
side. The nerves of the lower limb, which are
larger and thicker than nerves elsewhere, are eas-

ily shown by ultrasound. Acute injuries to these nerves show a complete or partial interruption of a continuously hyperechoic nerve trunk and an echoless or hypoechoic zone in the interrupted area [13]. Entrapment of the lower limb nerves is commonly seen, such as in piriformis syndrome

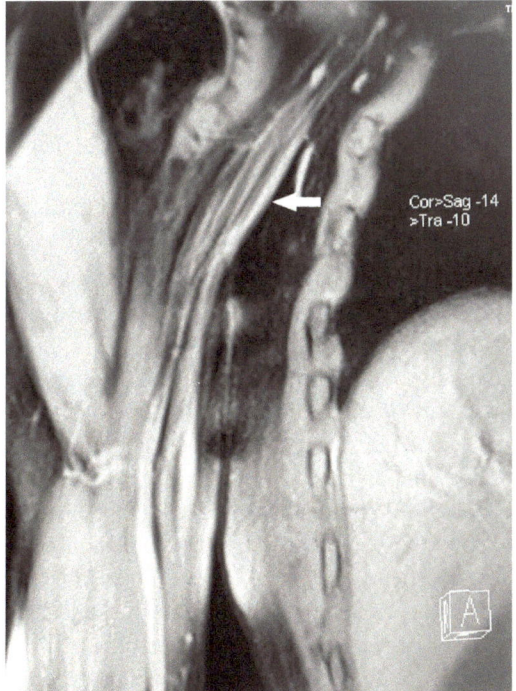

Fig. 4.161 MRI of nerve fibre fatty infiltration of the musculocutaneous nerve in the upper limb. Note: the yellow arrow is pointing to the nerve fibre fatty infiltration

and femoral lateral cutaneous nerve entrapment syndrome, which are both caused by blood circulation problems and demyelination due to repeated friction of peripheral nerves at locations with complex structures. The ultrasonic appearance of these injuries include the narrowing of the nerves at entrapment sites, with reduced or inhomogeneous echo, blurred and absent bundle structures, enlarged and increased echo in the epineurium and the distal end nerves at the entrapment site, as well as twisted and enlarged or unevenly swollen nerve ends.

4.3.1 Sciatic Nerve Injury (Cases 64–66)

Sciatic nerve lesions due to trauma, iatrogenic injury and fracture-inducing soft tissue lesions are commonly seen in the clinic, and these can cause functional impediments of the limbs, which affects patients' quality of life if they are not diagnosed early, if active and effective diagnosis and treatment are not provided, or if rehabilitation is poor. Relevant clinical symptoms include pain on the affected sides of the lower limbs, and in serious cases, walking impediments.

Case 64

A female patient aged 44 years. Main complaint: patient experienced pain in her left limb 2 weeks earlier, which worsened and was accompanied

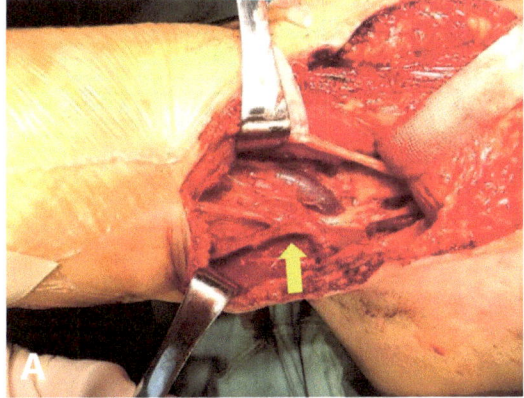
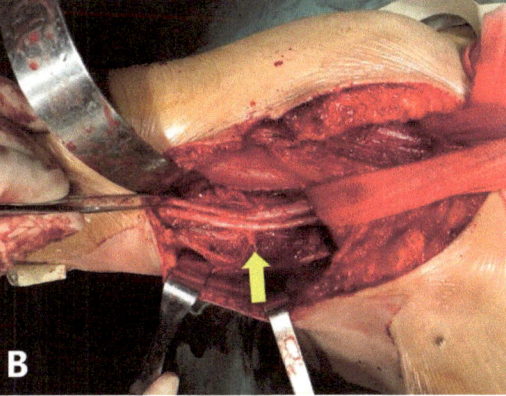

Fig. 4.162 Image of the operation for nerve fibre fatty infiltration of the musculocutaneous nerve in the upper limb at the axilla. (**a**): before debridement of nerve fibre fatty infiltration, (**b**): after debridement of nerve fibre fatty infiltration; the arrow is pointing to the exposed nerve after debridement

by restricted movements 5 days earlier. Current medical history: the patient experienced pain in her left lower limb without obvious causes 2 weeks prior. The pain worsened and was accompanied by restricted limb movements 5 days prior. Specialized physical examination: pressing pains (+) on the left hip and thigh; sensation: disappearance of skin sensation on the front and lateral sides of the crus and in the dorsal and bottom regions of the foot below the knee joint. Ultrasonic examination: the diameter of the left sciatic nerve that ran between the piriformis was 0.42 cm (contralateral side was 0.53 cm) at the piriformis outlet, with a reduced echo zone measuring 2.2 cm × 1.2 cm. Ultrasound finding: the left sciatic nerve ran continuously, with

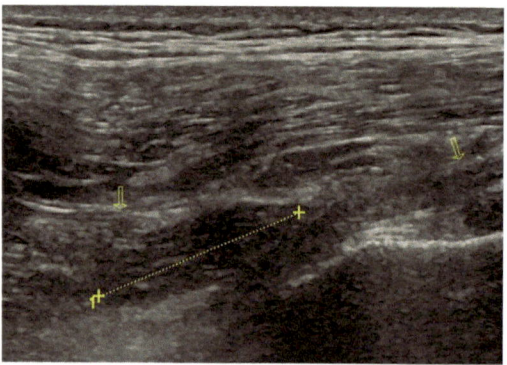

Fig. 4.163 Ultrasonogram of piriformis syndrome in the lower limb. Note: the arrow is pointing to the sciatic nerve and the piriformis is at the Vernier calliper

a hypoechoic piriformis, and demonstrated entrapment at the outlet; the injured nerve was thinner than the contralateral nerve, and thus piriformis syndrome was considered (Fig. 4.163) (Videos 4.58 and 4.59). The symptoms were eased after treatments involving antiphlogosis, pain release, and neural function repair.

ER 4.58 Dynamic image and explanation of piriformis syndrome

ER 4.59 Dynamic image and explanation of a normal contralateral piriformis

Case 65

A female patient aged 33 years. Main complaint: movement of the patient's left lower limb has been restricted for the past 10 years due to trauma. Current medical history: the patient suffered trauma-induced pain, bleeding, abnormal skin sensation, weak muscle force and a restricted ankle joint on her left lower limb 10 years earlier. Specialized physical examination: the patient had a limp along with drop and malformation of her left foot, amyotrophy (+) of the tibialis anterior, the peroneus longus and peroneus brevis muscles in her left leg; she also experienced hypaesthesia of the skin on the lateral part of her left leg and in the dorsal and bottom regions of her left foot by needling examination; the patient was also incapable of active extension of her left foot and toes and

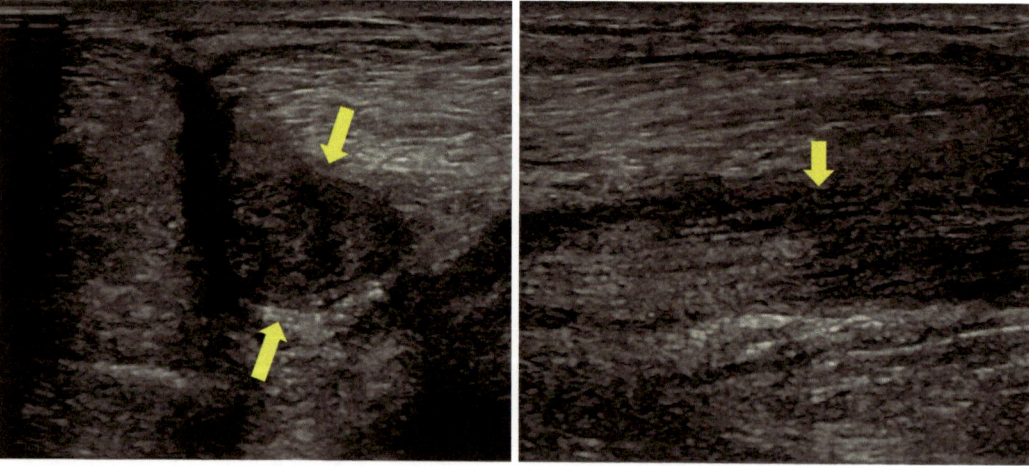

Fig. 4.164 Ultrasonogram of sciatic nerve injury and neuroma formation. Note: the yellow arrow is pointing to the short and long axes of an enlarged sciatic nerve and neuroma formation

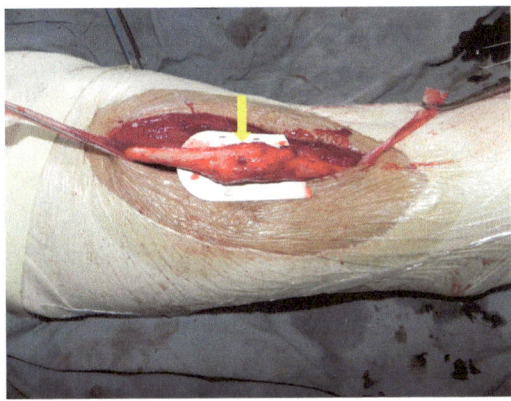

Fig. 4.165 Image of the operation for sciatic nerve injury and neuroma formation. Note: the yellow arrow is pointing to a neuroma of the sciatic nerve

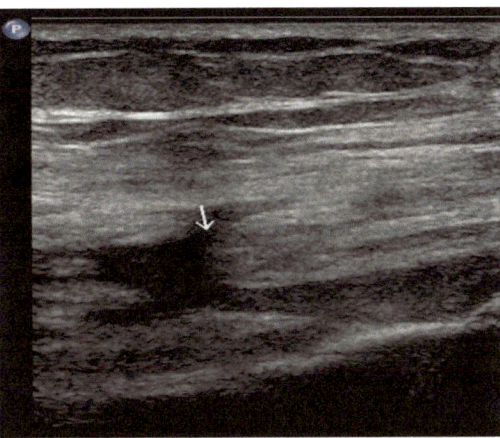

Fig. 4.166 Ultrasonogram of sciatic nerve fracture and the formation of traumatic neuroma. Note: the arrow is pointing to the sciatic nerve fracture

had 0-level muscle force of the left anterior tibial muscle and common extensor digitorum muscle, as well as reduction of muscle force of the adductor muscle in the left foot; patient had II-level muscle force of the peroneus longus and peroneus brevis muscles; patient experienced plantar flexion and a reduction of adductor muscle force of the left foot, and II-level muscle force of the triceps and posterior tibial muscle of the left crus; Tinel's sign (+) under the hip in the left lower limb.

Ultrasonic finding: part of the left sciatic nerve ran continuously and was enlarged and oedematous at the root of the thigh; the nerve demonstrated reduced echo and was 1.1 cm in diameter, 3.4 cm in length and 0.32 cm in diameter at the distal end. Ultrasound diagnosis: the left sciatic nerve ran continuously and was partially enlarged and oedematous at the root of the thigh, with reduced echo; thus, sciatic nerve injury was considered, and neuroma formation was suspected; alternatively, there could have been cohesion with the surrounding tissues (Figs. 4.164 and 4.165) (Video 4.60).

Operation: the sciatic nerve was enlarged and had obvious cohesion. Surgery should loosen the nerve and its cohesion with surrounding tissues. By five-minute high-voltage electrical stimulation, the epineurium along the nerve's path was completely loosened, and thus the cohesion to the surrounding was eliminated. Postoperative diagnosis: left sciatic nerve injury and neuroma formation.

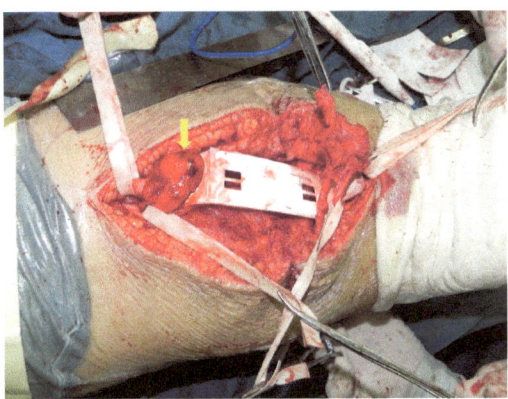

Fig. 4.167 Image of the operation for sciatic nerve fracture and the formation of traumatic neuroma. Note: the yellow arrow is pointing to the sciatic nerve fracture and the formation of traumatic neuroma

ER 4.60 Dynamic image and explanation of sciatic nerve injury and neuroma formation

Case 66
See (Figs. 4.166 and 4.167) (Video 4.61).

ER 4.61 Dynamic image and explanation of sciatic nerve fracture and the formation of traumatic neuroma

Summary Sciatic nerve injury is often associated with pain in the lower limbs. Therefore, sonographers should mainly observe whether the sciatic nerve runs continuously, is enlarged, is oedematous, has a fracture or if a neuroma is present.

Notes 1. Piriformis syndrome has clinical symptoms similar to those of slipped disc, and thus it requires careful identification; 2. The basis for identification is to understand the anatomy of the piriformis and sciatic nerve, comprehensive clinical symptoms and abnormal findings in the ultrasonogram; 3. For patients with similar symptoms, sonographers should offer valuable diagnostic information for clinical treatments as far as possible.

4.3.2 Peroneal Nerve Injury (Cases 67–70)

Peroneal nerve injury is a clinically common disease. The definite diagnosis is key for the determination of the surgical approach. The ultrasonic examination is conducive to fully understanding the types, ranges and quantities of peroneal nerve lesions, whose clinical features indicate different extents of common peroneal nerve injuries, i.e. numbness of the lateral parts of the legs and dorsal feet, restrictions when the feet are lifted, and a positive electromyogram.

Case 67

Main complaint: the movements of the right knee joint had been restricted for 4 months. Current medical history: the patient accidentally injured the right knee joint, suffered pain and later walking functional impairment; consequently, the injured limb had to be lifted high when walking, and dorsal stretch and eversion were confined. Specialized physical examination: limp during walking because the right lower limb had to be lifted high when walking, without obvious abnormality in sensation of the right leg; II-level muscle force of the right tibialis anterior muscle, extensor pollicis longus and peroneus longus and peroneus brevis muscles.

Ultrasound finding: the right common peroneal nerve ran continuously but was partially enlarged to 0.8 cm in diameter at the capitula fibula with a reduced echo (the normal part nerve is 0.26 cm in diameter). Ultrasound diagnosis: the right common peroneal nerve ran continuously and was enlarged at the capitula fibula, with a

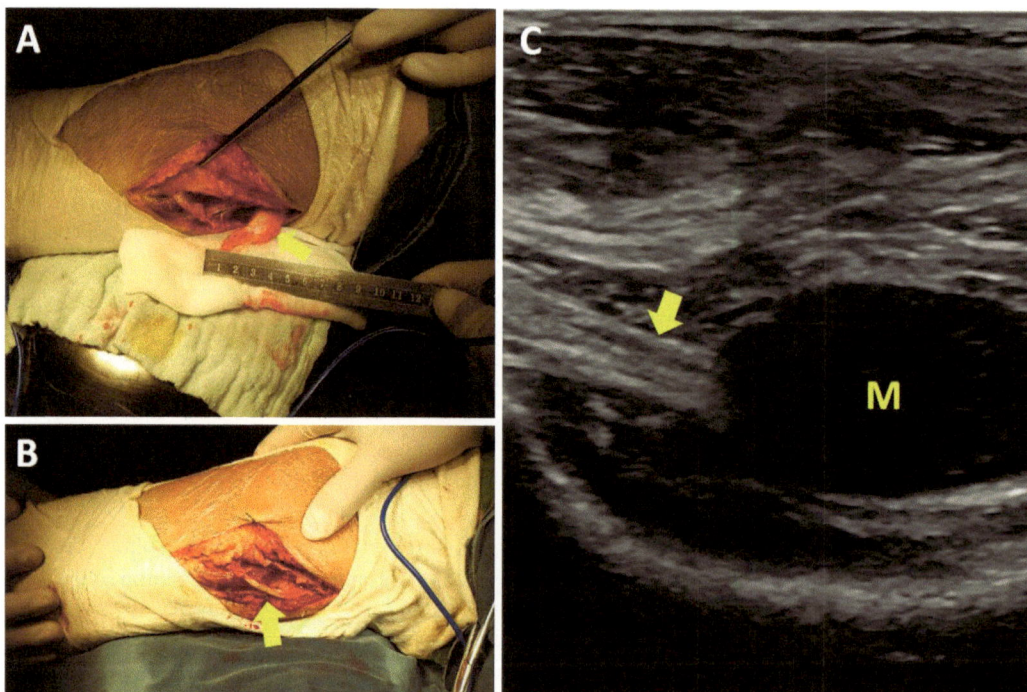

Fig. 4.168 Ultrasonogram and image of the operation for common peroneal nerve injury. Note: the yellow arrow in (**a**) is pointing to neuroma formation (before repair) due to common peroneal nerve injury; the yellow arrow in (**b**) is pointing to the repaired common peroneal nerve; the yellow arrow in (**c**) is pointing to the common peroneal nerve and M is the neuroma

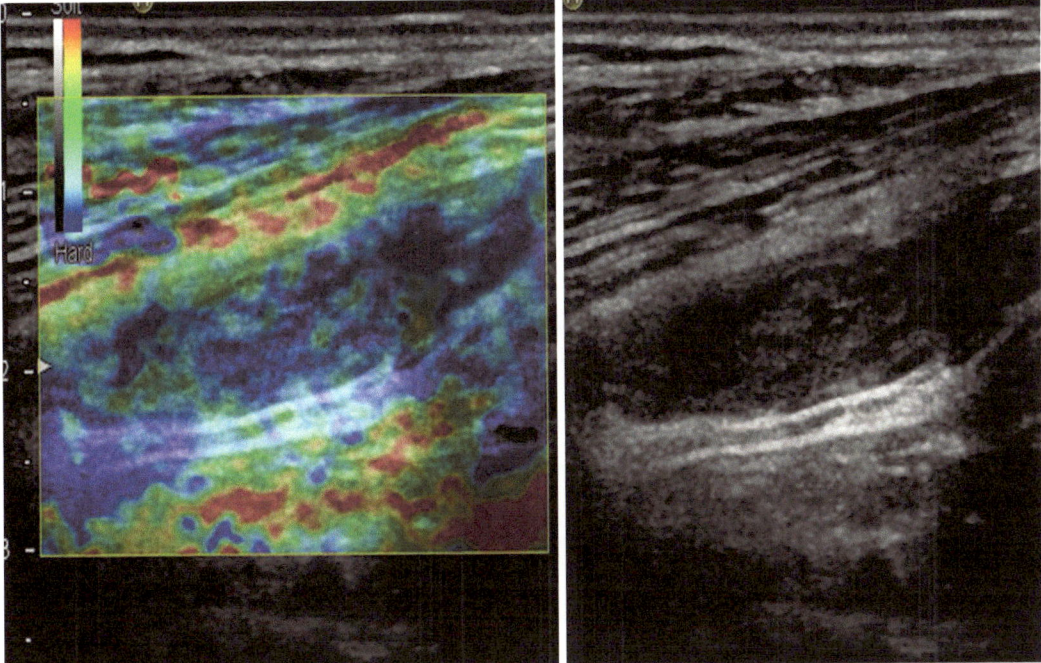

Fig. 4.169 Elastosonography for common peroneal nerve injury. Note: the blue area in the left figure is the zone of common peroneal nerve injury; the right figure shows the 2D ultrasonogram

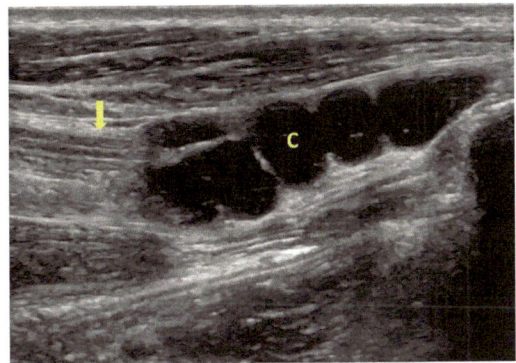

Fig. 4.170 Ultrasonogram of common peroneal nerve injury. Note: the yellow arrow is pointing to the common peroneal nerve and C indicates the formation of a cyst

reduced echo, and thus common peroneal nerve injury was considered (Figs. 4.168 and 4.169) (Video 4.62).

Operation: during surgery, part of the common peroneal nerve stretching across the capitula fibula was enlarged, pale and was under high tension. By further exploration, its inner capitula fibula was squeezed and expanded. After incising its periosteum, the cartilage below it had a lesion and overgrowth. When the lesion was scraped off using a

special spoon, the tension of the common peroneal nerve was reduced. By scanning the distal end, the surrounding bundles at the outlet of the common peroneal nerve became compressed, but after loosening it, the tension of the common peroneal nerve was reduced and a portion of it was restored.

ER 4.62 Dynamic image and explanation of common peroneal nerve injury

Case 68
See (Fig. 4.170) (Video 4.63).

ER 4.63 Dynamic image and explanation of common peroneal nerve injury

Case 69
See (Figs. 4.171 and 4.172) (Videos 4.64 and 4.65).

ER 4.64 Dynamic image and explanation of common peroneal nerve compression

ER 4.65 Explanation of common peroneal nerve compression during surgery

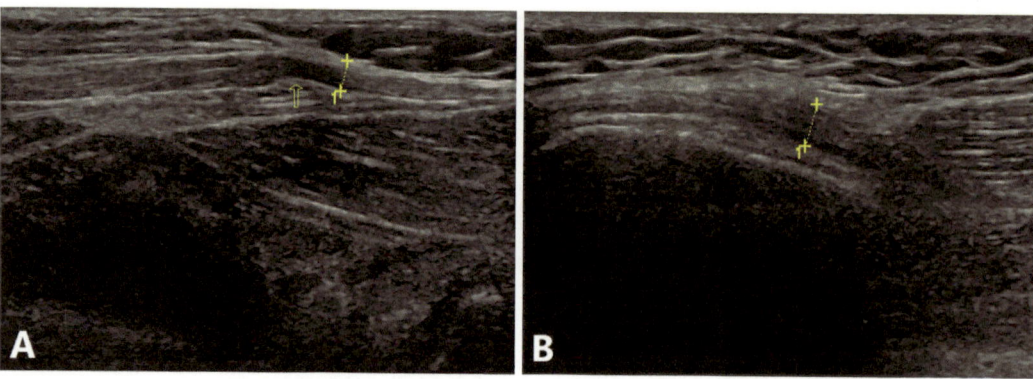

Fig. 4.171 Ultrasonogram of common peroneal nerve compression. Note: (**a**): common peroneal nerve compression (arrows), (**b**): the calliper indicates common peroneal nerve oedema

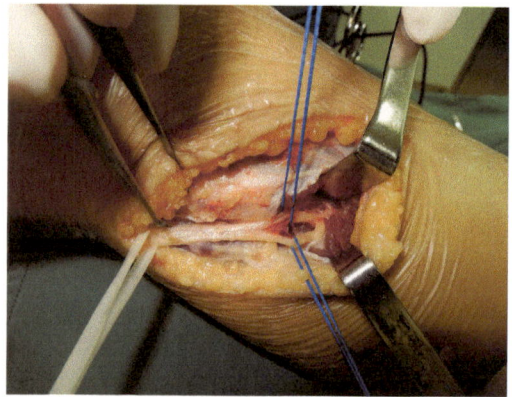

Fig. 4.172 Image of the operation for common peroneal nerve compression

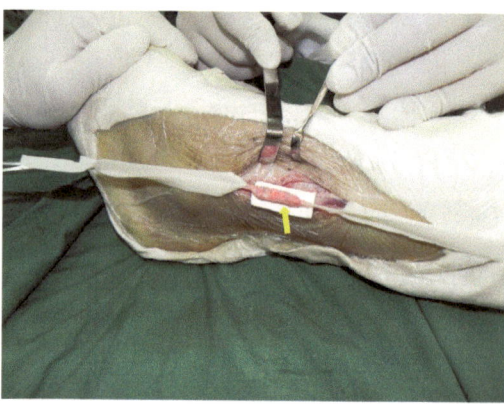

Fig. 4.174 Image of the operation for traumatic neuroma of the superficial peroneal nerve above the lateral malleolus. Note: the yellow arrow is pointing to the traumatic neuroma of the superficial peroneal nerve

Case 70
See (Figs. 4.173 and 4.174).

Summary Notes: 1. The most commonly seen common peroneal nerve injury is entrapment at the capitula fibula and on the plane formed by the convergence of the common peroneal nerve and the tibial nerve; 2. Clinical features include the incapability for dorsal flexure of the ankles; 3. When patients exhibit the above symptoms, sonographers should observe the path of the common peroneal nerve and the superficial peroneal nerve, especially at the specific positions mentioned above.

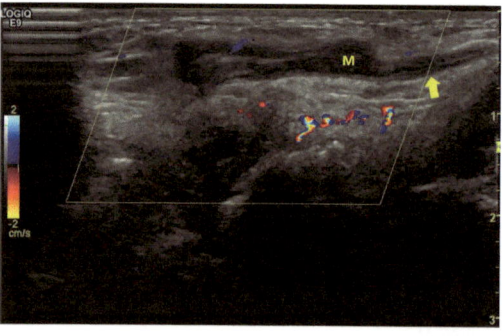

Fig. 4.173 Ultrasonogram of a traumatic neuroma of the superficial peroneal nerve above the lateral malleolus. Note: the arrow is pointing to the superficial peroneal nerve, and M is the traumatic neuroma of the superficial peroneal nerve

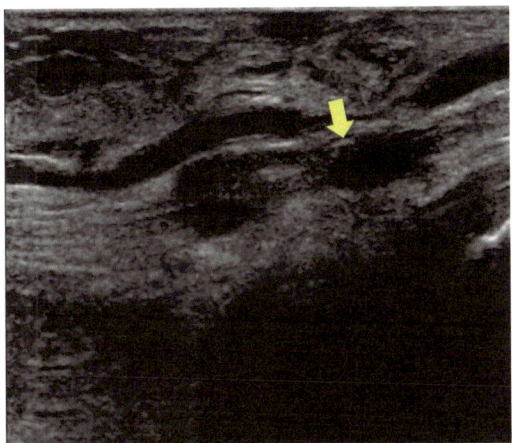

Fig. 4.175 Ultrasonogram of tarsal tunnel syndrome. Note: the yellow arrow is pointing to the enlarged nerve with oedema

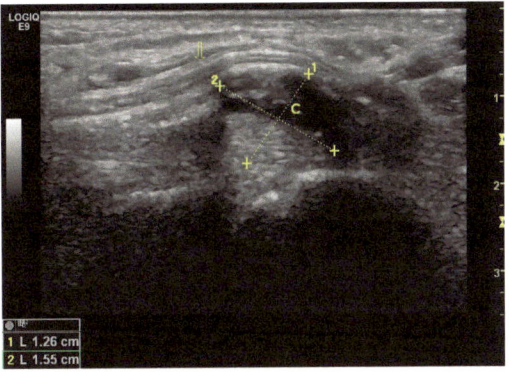

Fig. 4.177 Ultrasonogram of tibial nerve injury (extra-neural cyst) at the medial malleolus. Note: the yellow arrow is pointing to the tibial nerve, and the Vernier calliper indicates the formation of an extraneural cyst due to tibial nerve injury

ER 4.66 Dynamic image and explanation of tibial nerve injury and cyst formation at the medial malleolus

Summary Tibial nerve injury is often manifested as tarsal tunnel syndrome and tarsal tunnel entrapment due to extraneural cyst formation. When patients suffer numbness at the heels, sonographers should scan the tibial nerve at the medial malleolus to observe whether there is entrapment due to an extraneural cyst.

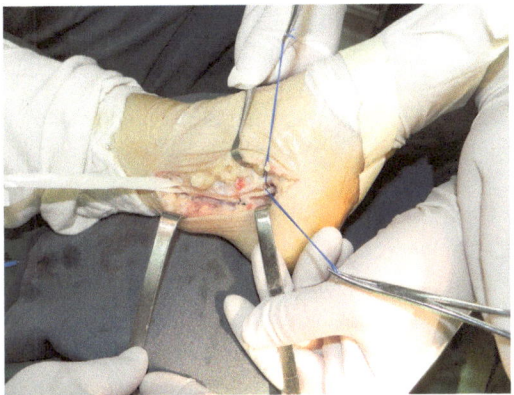

Fig. 4.176 Image of the operation for tarsal tunnel syndrome

4.3.4 Schwannoma of Peripheral Nerves of the Lower Limb (Cases 73–76)

Schwannoma often occurs in adults in the form of a single tumour covering a large area of the body, especially in the neck and limbs. Peripheral schwannoma needs to be distinguished from neurofibroma, swollen lymph nodes, haemangioma and abscess.

4.3.3 Tibial Nerve Injury (Cases 71–72)

The tibial nerve controls the skin on the lateral posterior side of the lower half of the crus, lateral ankle, the lateral edge of the feet to the little toes and sole of the foot. Tibial nerve injury will cause numbness, pain and impairments in sensation and movement in the corresponding controlled areas.

Case 71
See (Figs. 4.175 and 4.176).

Case 72
See (Figs. 4.177 and 4.178) (Video 4.66).

Case 73
A male patient aged 38 years. Main complaint: a large mass gradually grew at the front, medial side of his upper left thigh, along with pain in the inner side of the thigh for 5 years. Current medical history: the patient incidentally discovered a mass on the internal side of his upper left thigh without obvious causes 5 years ago, along with

Fig. 4.178 Image of the operation for tibial nerve injury (extraneural cyst) at the medial malleolus. Note: (**a**) is the diagram before the decollement of an extraneural cyst that formed due to tibial nerve injury, and (**b**) is the diagram after the decollement of an extraneural cyst that formed due to tibial nerve injury

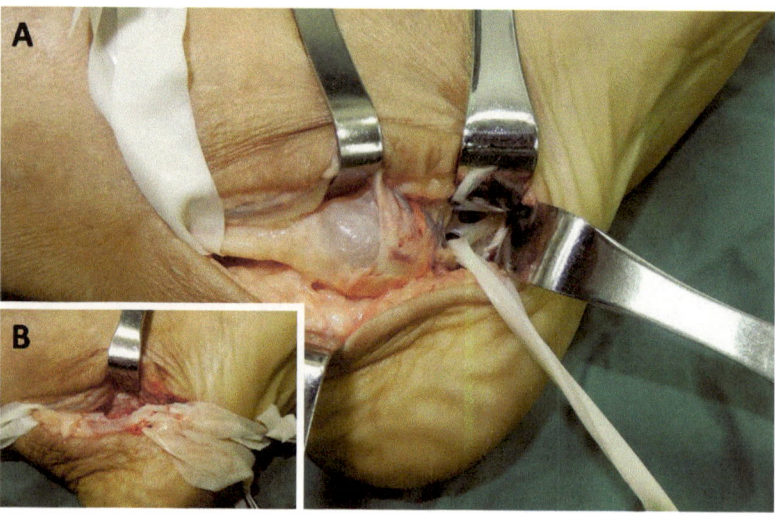

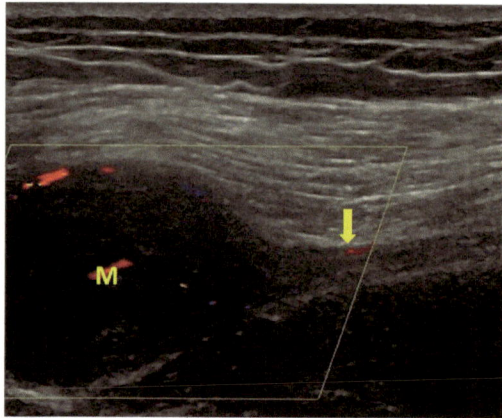

Fig. 4.179 Ultrasonogram of a femoral nerve schwannoma. Note: the yellow arrow is pointing to the femoral nerve and M is the femoral nerve schwannoma

local pressing pain. He once underwent treatment for rheumatic arthritis at a local hospital, and later the pain worsened, especially at night, and even affected his daily life.

Ultrasound finding: a mixed mass 4.3 × 5.4 cm in size in the inner muscular layer of the left thigh, with both ends connecting to the femoral nerve; thus, schwannoma was considered (Figs. 4.179 and 4.180) (Video 4.67). Operation: a mass 6.0 cm × 3.0 cm in size was observed in the femoral nerve in the inner muscular layer of the left thigh, with a clear boundary and available mobility. After careful separation and incision of the membrane enveloping the mass, it was found that the mass was derived from the bundle branch

of the femoral nerve and fat-like and light yellow in appearance with clear fluid inside. It was then confirmed to be a femoral nerve schwannoma.

ER 4.67 Dynamic image and explanation of femoral nerve schwannoma

Case 74

A female patient aged 64 years. Main complaint: a mass was found in the right popliteal space 14 years earlier, and over the past 3 years, the pain caused by the mass had worsened. Current medical history: the patient found a mass in her right popliteal space without apparent cause 14 years ago, along with discontinuous pain but no other symptoms. Over the past 3 years, the pain worsened and was accompanied by numbness of the right lower limb and radiating pain. Specialized physical examination: a hard mass 1.0 cm × 0.5 cm in size and with a blurred boundary could be palpated at the right popliteal space; available mobility, a smooth surface, pressing pain (+) and posterior pain radiating to her leg and toes were also observed. On the right side, Tinel's sign (+) was found. MRI performed at another hospital: due to abnormal signals in soft tissues in the right popliteal space, a cyst was considered.

Ultrasonic finding: there was a hypoechoic zone 1.3 cm × 0.8 cm in size in the path of the common peroneal nerve at the right popliteal space, with a clear boundary, regular form and connection to

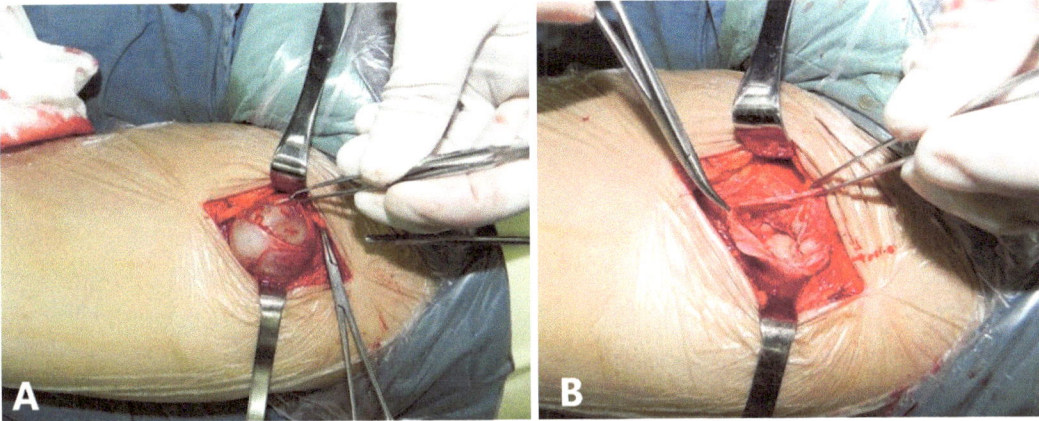

Fig. 4.180 Image of the operation for femoral nerve schwannoma. Note: (**a**) is before the decollement of femoral nerve schwannoma, (**b**) is after the decollement of femoral nerve schwannoma

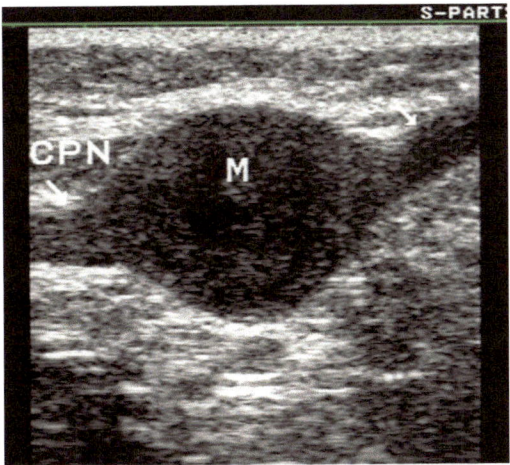

Fig. 4.181 Ultrasonogram of a common peroneal nerve schwannoma. Note: the yellow arrow is pointing to the common peroneal nerve and M is the schwannoma

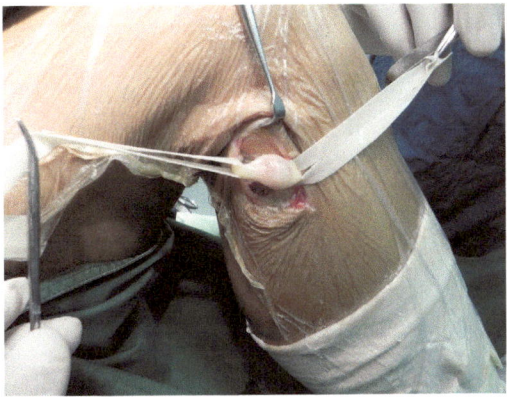

Fig. 4.182 Image of the operation for common peroneal nerve schwannoma

the common peroneal nerve. Ultrasound diagnosis: common peroneal nerve schwannoma in the right popliteal space (Figs. 4.181 and 4.182).

Operation: during surgery, a hard mass 1 cm in diameter that was round and greyish yellow in colour was found in the epineurium of the common peroneal nerve, with total exposure of its neural proximal and distal ends. After the incision of the epineurium, the mass was separated thoroughly by cutting off the fine neural bundle branches that were connected to the mass, without damaging the common peroneal nerve.

Pathological examination: cellular schwannoma of the common peroneal nerve (right popliteal space).

Case 75

A male patient aged 42 years. Main complaint: the patient began to experience discontinuous pain and discomfort at the posterior proximal end of his right crus 3 years earlier, especially when he squatted and was exhausted, but the pain was relieved after rest or simple movements. Specialized physical examination: a mass could be palpated at the posterior proximal end of his right crus. His right knee joint had good mobility. MRI performed at another hospital: schwannoma at the rear edge of the posterior tibial tendon of the right crus was likely.

Ultrasonic finding: there was a hypoechoic zone 3.5 cm × 1.9 cm in size that connected to the tibial nerve with a clear boundary and

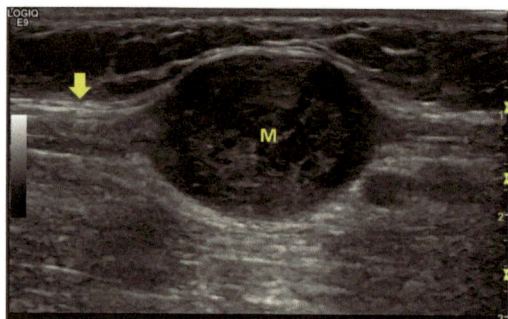

Fig. 4.183 Ultrasonogram of a tibial nerve schwannoma. Note: the yellow arrow is pointing to the tibial nerve, and M is the schwannoma

a regular shape. Ultrasound diagnosis: a solid mass was observed in the posterior tibial muscular layer of the right crus, and thus schwannoma of the tibial nerve was initially considered (Fig. 4.183) (Video 4.68).

Operation: a mass 4 cm × 2 cm in size was observed in the epineurium of the tibial nerve during surgery. After the incision of the epineurium, the mass was completed removed.

Pathologic findings: plexiform schwannomas (right crus).

ER 4.68 Dynamic image and explanation of schwannoma of the tibial nerve

Case 76
See (Figs. 4.184 and 4.185) (Video 4.69).

ER 4.69 Dynamic image and explanation of tibial nerve schwannoma at the medial malleolus

Summary Schwannoma in the lower limbs is similar to Schwannoma in the upper limbs. When a mass with a reticulate structure is present in the popliteal space, the continuity of nerves should be determined, and the relationships between mixed lumps and nerves should be established.

Notes The ultrasonogram might show if the mass is solid, mixed or cystic, and thus during scanning, the relationship between the mass and its surrounding nerves should be considered.

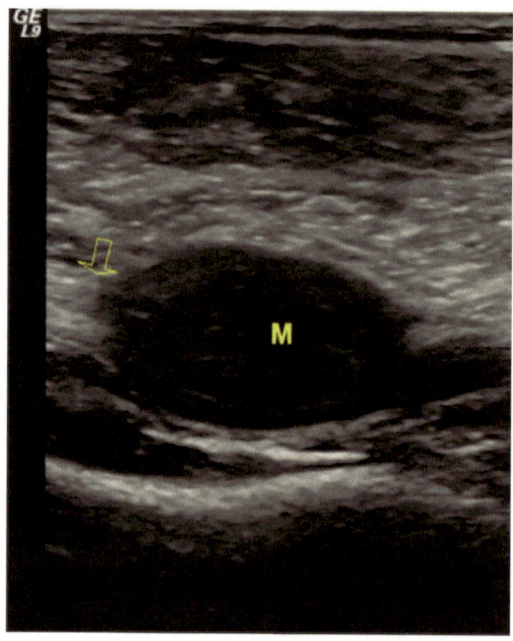

Fig. 4.184 Ultrasonogram of a tibial nerve schwannoma at the medial malleolus. Note: the arrow is pointing to the tibial nerve, and M is the schwannoma

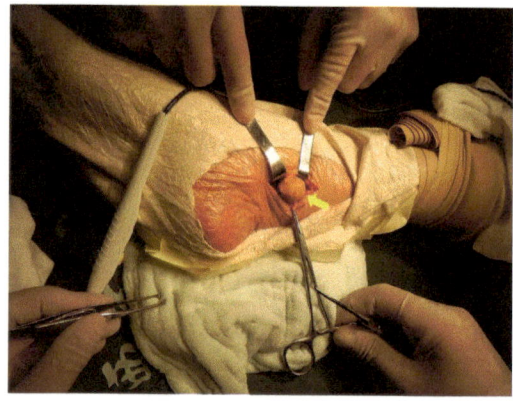

Fig. 4.185 Image of the operation for tibial nerve schwannoma at the medial malleolus. Note: the yellow arrow is pointing to the tibial nerve schwannoma

4.3.5 Cystic Degeneration and Fibromatosis of the Sciatic Nerve (Cases 77–78)

Case 77
See (Fig. 4.186) (Video 4.70).

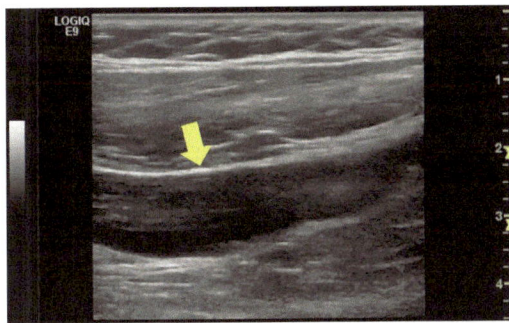

Fig. 4.186 Ultrasonogram of cystic degeneration of the sciatic nerve. Note: the yellow arrow is pointing to cystic degeneration of the sciatic nerve

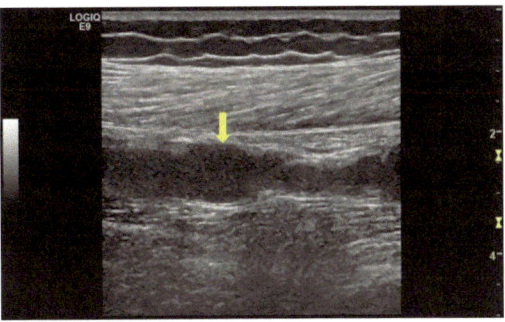

Fig. 4.187 Ultrasonogram of neurofibromatosis of the sciatic nerve. Note: the yellow arrow is pointing to the enlarged hypoechoic sciatic nerve

ER 4.70 Dynamic image and explanation of cystic degeneration of the sciatic nerve

Case 78

A male patient aged 32 years. The patient visited the hospital for diagnosis and treatment because his left lower limb had sensation and active movement impairment for the past year. An MRI examination performed at another hospital revealed multiple cystic abnormal signals in the fat tissue space among the posterior muscle groups at the middle and lower parts of his left thigh, and varicosity was suspected. Therefore, the patient was advised to undergo further examination. The ultrasound performed in our department showed an abnormal echo in his left sciatic nerve, and thus a CEUS examination was immediately performed. Contrast agent perfusion was shown in the abnormal echo zone, and thus neurofibromatosis was considered (Figs. 4.187 and 4.188) (Video 4.71).

ER 4.71 Dynamic image and explanation of CEUS of neurofibromatosis in the sciatic nerve

Summary The two cases discussed above warn us that if the ultrasonic examination shows cystic or hypo-echo in the tubular structure that runs along the nerve, it should not be assumed that it is a blood vessel or a cyst. Observation of the paths of the blood vessel and nerve is required, and CEUS, which can show the appearance of

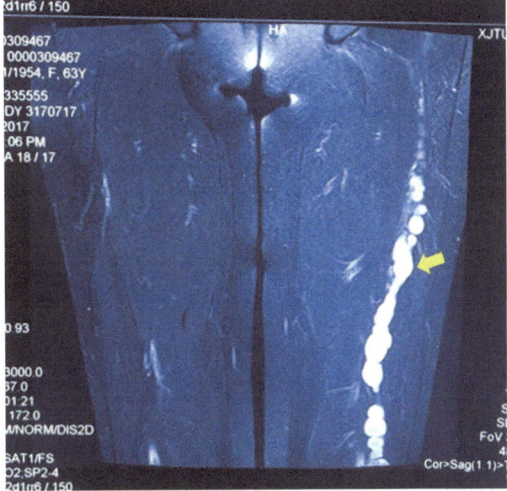

Fig. 4.188 MRI of neurofibromatosis of the sciatic nerve. Note: the hyperintense zone indicated by the yellow arrow is neurofibromatosis of the sciatic nerve

contrast agent signals with blood supply in the nerves, can be used for identification and diagnosis.

4.3.6 Multiple *Neurofibromatosis* Throughout the Entire Body (Cases 79)

Neurofibromatosis (NF), also known as multiple neurofibroma, is a type of *neurocutaneous syndrome* and is an autosomal dominant disease with multisystem abnormalities due to abnormal neural crest cell differentiation. This disorder generally involves nerves, muscles, bones, viscera and skin and has an incidence rate of 3/100,000. It is accompanied by characteristic moles and spots on the skin, and therefore, it is also called *phakomatoses*, which is a congenital disease resulting from maldevelopment. Nearly 15–20% of NF patients experience central nervous system tumours or other malignant tumours. According to the clinical features and genetic locations, NF can be divided into neurofibromatosis type I (NFI) and neurofibromatosis type II (NFII).

Subcutaneous neurofibromatosis, which is a common symptom of NF, grows as solitary different-sized nodules or beads in a quantity of ten or even more than one thousand. These cover a large area of the body, especially the lower limbs, and the larger nodules droop similar to a pouch due to gravity. Over 90% of patients have multiple tumours less than 3 mm in diameter and dark-brown skin due to pigmentation. These spots are termed café-au-lait-spots, which do not protrude from the surface of normal skin, but rather, they protrude from abnormal areas on which hairs may be growing. In addition, some other diseases may also develop, such as connective tissue disease, skeletal deformities, tumours or malformation of the central nervous system; other diseases that can develop include enlargement of some organs, such as giant epityphlon malformation and macrodactylia. In all, 30% of patients with neurofibromatosis may suffer from bony defects, scoliosis, depressed skull, pseudarthrosis in the tibia and other bone changes. Such tumours often grow in the cranium or in the spinal cavity and lead to compression symptoms, such as intracranial hypertension, paralysis and paraesthesia.

Case 79

A male patient aged 10 years. Multiple cafe-au-lait spots were observed over the body and limbs, along with weakness in the upper limbs. The ultrasonic examination performed at a local hospital suggested possible swollen lymph nodes in the neck. Further ultrasound examination at our hospital led to a diagnosis of neurofibromatosis of the neck and upper and lower limbs (Figs. 4.189, 4.190, 4.191, 4.192, 4.193 and 4.194) (Video 4.72).

ER 4.72 Dynamic image and explanation of whole-body neurofibromatosis

Summary Such cases are special in appearance. If the typical cafe-au-lait spots occur on the skin, observing whether the nerves are abnormal should be considered first.

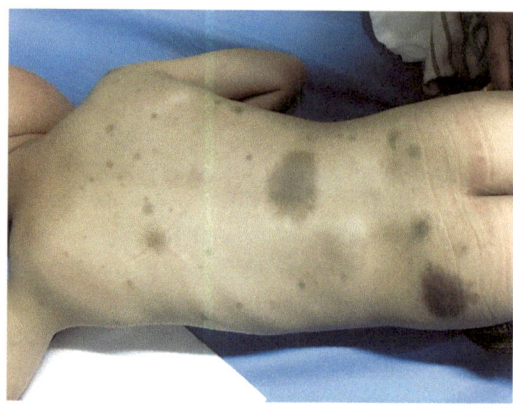

Fig. 4.189 External view of whole-body multiple cafe-au-lait spots

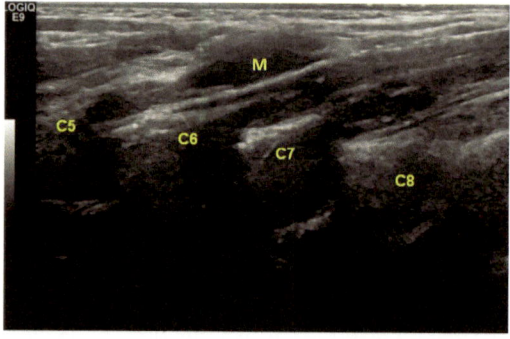

Fig. 4.190 Ultrasonogram of whole-body neurofibromatosis (involving the brachial plexus). Note: C5, C6, C7 and C8 are the roots of the brachial plexus, and M is neurofibromatosis

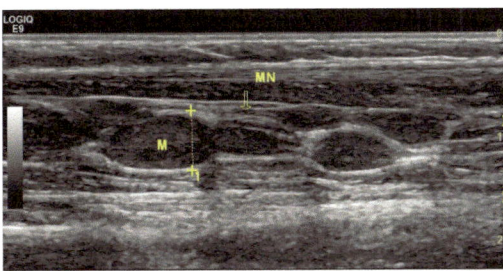

Fig. 4.191 Ultrasonogram of whole-body neurofibromatosis (involving the median nerve). Note: MN is the median nerve and M is neurofibromatosis

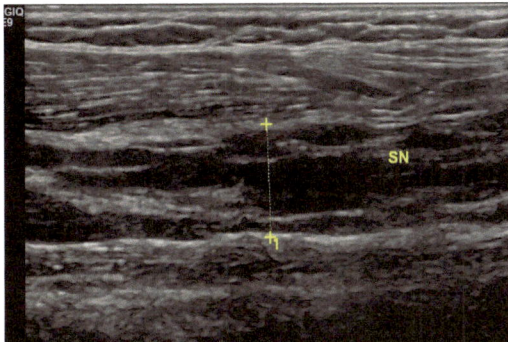

Fig. 4.192 Ultrasonogram of whole-body neurofibromatosis (involving the sciatic nerve). Note: SN is the sciatic nerve, and the Vernier calliper indicates the enlarged sciatic nerve with neurofibromatosis

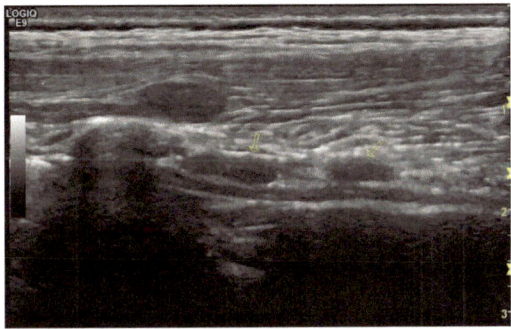

Fig. 4.193 Ultrasonogram of whole-body neurofibromatosis (involving the intercostal nerve). Note: the arrow is pointing to the neurofibromatosis of the intercostal nerve

Notes Patients often present to a hospital for diagnosis of masses or swollen lymph nodes. The ultrasound examination should encompass the

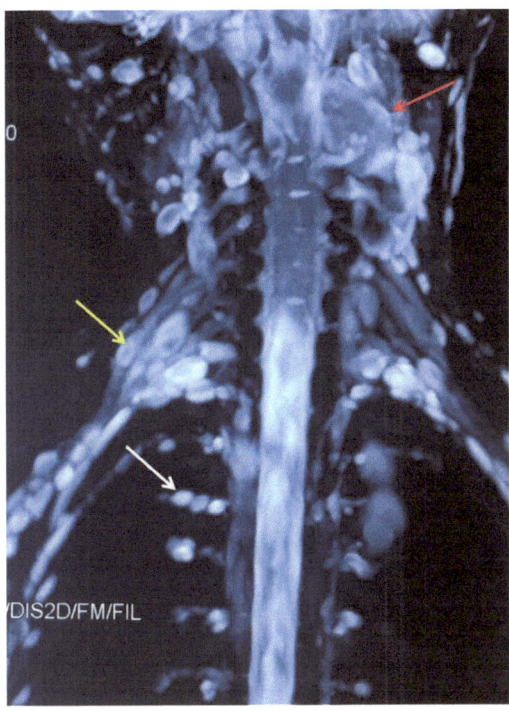

Fig. 4.194 MRI of whole-body neurofibromatosis. Note: the red arrow is pointing to the neurofibromatosis of the vagus nerve at the neck, the yellow arrow is pointing to the neurofibromatosis of the brachial plexus at the bundle level, and the white arrow is pointing to the neurofibromatosis of the intercostal nerve

scanning of major neural areas such as the brachial plexus at the neck and limbs to identify the mass as a tumour, lymph nodes or nerve fibres.

References

1. Snoj Ž, Riegler G, Moritz T, et al. Brachial plexus ultrasound in a patient with myelodysplastic syndrome and myelosarcoma. Muscle Nerve. 2017;56(6):E170–2.
2. Chen DZ, Cong R, Zheng MJ, et al. Differential diagnosis between pre- and postganglionic adult traumatic brachial plexus lesions by ultrasonography. Ultrasound Med Biol. 2011;37(8):1196–203.
3. Yeap LP, Liang YW, Nakashima H, et al. Impact of keyboard typing on the morphological changes of the median nerve. J Occup Health. 2017;59(5): 408–17.
4. Cartwright MS, Baute V, Caress JB, et al. Ultrahigh-frequency ultrasound of fascicles in the median nerve at the wrist. Muscle Nerve. 2017;56(4):819–22.

5. Nogueira-Barbosa MH, Lugão HB, Gregio-Júnior E, et al. Ultrasound elastography assessment of the median nerve in leprosy patients. Muscle Nerve. 2017;56(3):393–8.

6. Soldado F, Bertelli JA, Ghizoni MF. High median nerve injury: motor and sensory nerve transfers to restore function. Hand Clin. 2016;32(2):209–17.

7. Schuhfried O, Herceg M, Pieber K, et al. Interrater repeatability of motor nerve conduction velocity of the ulnar nerve. Am J Phys Med Rehabil. 2017;96(1):45–9.

8. Sallam AA, El-Deeb MS, Imam MA. Nerve transfer versus nerve graft for reconstruction of high ulnar nerve injuries. J Hand Surg Am. 2017;42(4):265–73.

9. Cook S, Gaston RG, Lourie GM. Ulnar nerve tendon transfers for pinch. Hand Clin. 2016;32(3):369–76.

10. Desai MJ, Daly CA, Seiler JG, et al. Radial to axillary nerve transfers: a combined case series. J Hand Surg Am. 2016;41(12):1128–34.

11. Cheah AE, Etcheson J, Yao J. Radial nerve tendon transfers. Hand Clin. 2016;32(3):323–38.

12. Song X, Abzug JM. Congenital radial nerve palsy. J Hand Surg Am. 2015;40(1):163–5.

13. Tubbs RS, Collin PG, D'Antoni AV, et al. Sciatic nerve intercommunications: new finding. World Neurosurg. 2017;98:176–81.

Application and Prospects of New Ultrasonic Technologies in the Diagnosis and Treatment of Peripheral Nerve Disorders

5

Minjuan Zheng, Dingzhang Chen, and Jing Wang

5.1 Application of Elastography to Peripheral Nerves

Ultrasonic elastography is an emerging non-invasive ultrasonic detection technology. Elasticity is an important physical characteristic of human tissue. In cases where a probe is used to press the peripheral nerves along the vertical (axial) direction, the nerves will become displaced, which is termed elastic strain; imaging by ultrasonic elastography utilizes the difference in colour codes to embody the differences in tissue elasticity, where softer tissues have a small elasticity modulus and are indicated by a red colour when they are pressed; in contrast, harder tissues have a large elasticity modulus and are indicated by a blue colour when they are pressed, and those tissues with medium hardness are indicated by a green colour [1, 2].

The boundaries of ordinary ultrasonic evaluation of peripheral nerve injury lie in clearly and intuitively displaying the distribution, paths, structures, lesion ranges and accurate location of peripheral nerves. When the peripheral nerves suffer mild, nontypical injuries or inflammatory infiltration, ordinary 2D ultrasonic scanning of the neural tissue interface may show unapparent changes in acoustic impedance differences and acoustic scattering coefficients. However, the elastic strain (hardness) of the injured nerves may have already changed and worsened with prolonged injury time (such as the formation of scars) (Figs. 5.1 and 5.2).

Shear-wave elasticity imaging, a type of ultrasound elastography, is also an emerging ultrasonic technology. Here, a probe is used to launch a safe acoustic radiation pulse into tissues at different depths, and thus a shear wave is generated by the efficient vibration of tissue particles at the locations pulsed. The generated shear wave, a kind of transverse wave, has a propagation velocity of 1–10 m/s in living tissues, and thus a rapid imaging system of 20,000 frames/s can be utilized to capture and track shear waves for real-time elastography. Obtaining the propagation velocity of tracked shear waves will acquire Young's modulus—the larger its value, the faster the shear wave speed and the harder the tissue. As the propagation velocity of shear waves is different in different tissues, real-time shear waves have been widely applied in the examination of solid organs such as the thyroid, breast, liver, spleen and kidney. In some studies, shear wave elastography was used to evaluate fibrosis or scarring of peripheral nerves, the changes in neural texture due to neural entrapment and neural inflammation, and the texture of neurogenic tumours. This indicates that shear wave elastography is valuable for early

M. Zheng (✉) · D. Chen · J. Wang
Department of Ultrasound, Xijing Hospital,
Fourth Military Medical University,
Xi'an, Shaanxi, China

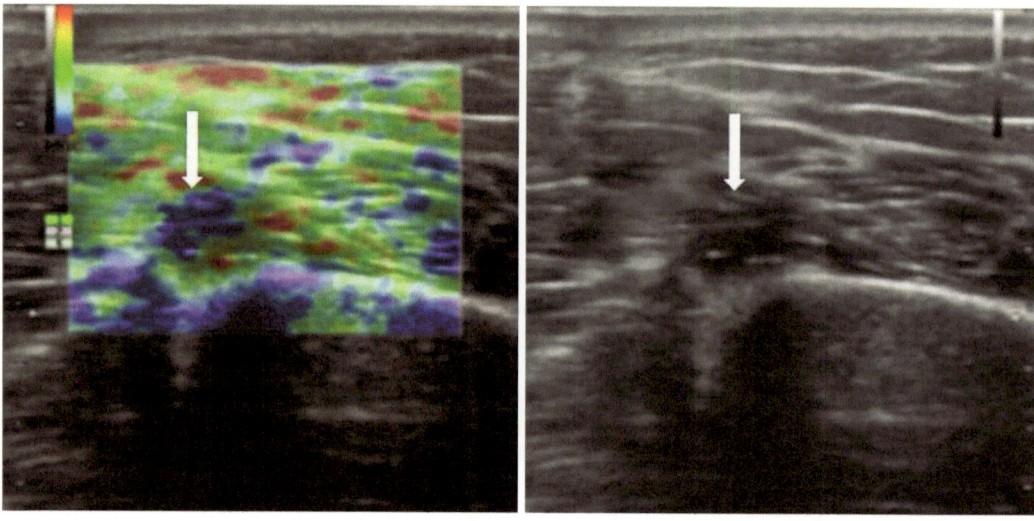

Fig. 5.1 Radial nerve fracture and scar formation. Note: the *arrow* indicates the radial nerve scar with increased hardness; the RTE rating is 4

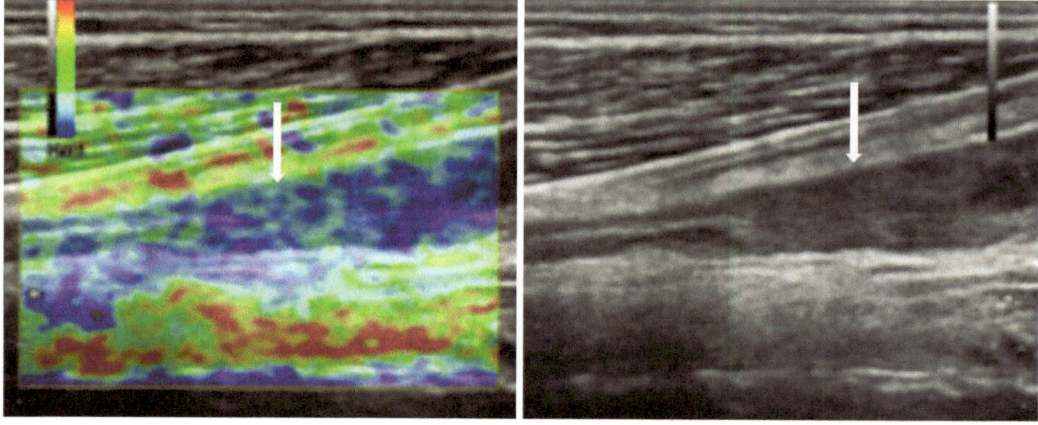

Fig. 5.2 Common peroneal nerve injury and neuroma formation. Note: at the arrow is the common peroneal nerve neuroma with higher hardness, and RTE rating is 5

diagnosis of neural lesions, but further technical improvements and studies are still needed.

5.2 Application of Contrast-Enhanced Ultrasonography in Peripheral Nerves

Contrast-enhanced ultrasonography (CEUS), which is based on an ordinary ultrasonic examination, is performed to observe the real-time microvascular perfusion of tissues according to the scattered signals of blood flow enhanced by the intravenous injection of ultrasonic contrast agent, to strengthen the judgement, sensitivity and specificity of ultrasonic diagnosis. This modality can provide more information on blood flow in solid tissues, and it can reflect differences in blood perfusion between normal and pathological tissues. Therefore, it can raise the detection rate of ultrasonic diagnosis and identify both benign and malignant lesions. CEUS examination can be performed quickly (in approximately 5–8 min) with no need for a skin test, as it involves no ionizing radiation and no liver or kidney toxicity.

CEUS has already been widely applied for examination of superficial organs, abdominal organs and the cardiovascular system, as well as for neuroimaging. The diagnoses of some cases described above were confirmed by CEUS (Figs. 5.3 and 5.4). Some studies indicated that peripheral nerve injuries at different stages show different CEUS features. In the early stage (within 1 week), granulation tissue has yet to be formed. Due to the fracture of small vessels at the broken end, the blood effuses to the surrounding area and forms a fresh haematocele (anechoic zone). The ruptured small vessels in the perineurium or epineurium are still not occluded, and thus the contrast agent usually encounters the fresh haematocele. In the middle and late stages (more than 1 week), granulation tissue or scar has been formed. Since the newly generated vessels in the

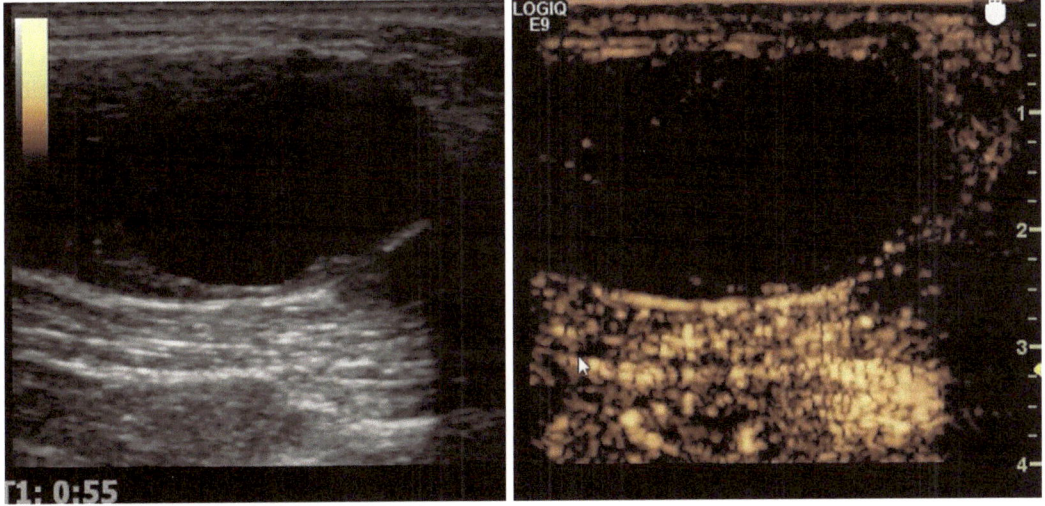

Fig. 5.3 CEUS of cystic degeneration of a brachial plexus schwannoma

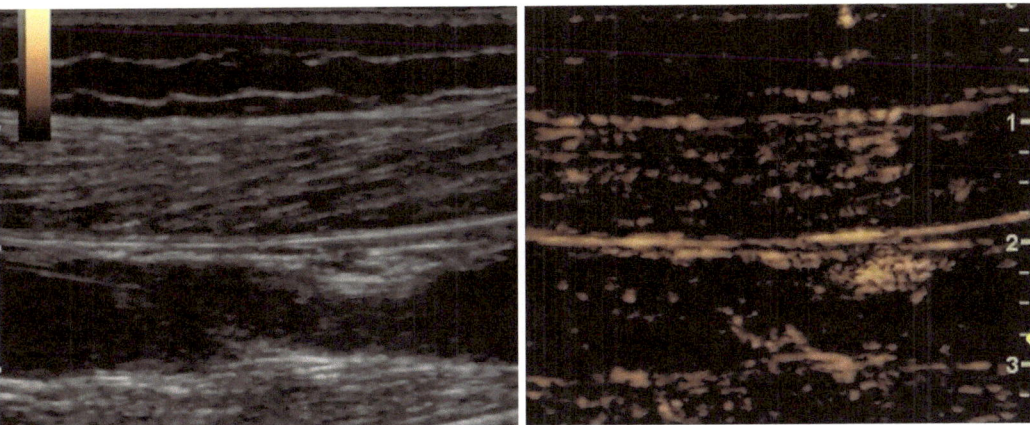

Fig. 5.4 CEUS of sciatic nerve neurofibromatosis

hyperplastic granulation tissue are thin and irregular, CEUS shows inhomogeneous low enhancement. Finally, a few months later, the regenerated axons at the broken end grow in all directions are irregularly and thus a traumatic neuroma is formed. The vessels are totally occluded, and no contrast agent can enter.

CEUS for peripheral nerve injury at different stages is a reminder of the importance of the avoidance of delay in surgery timing due to the formation of scars and the observation and evaluation of postoperative effects. CEUS can perform accurate and non-invasive diagnosis of peripheral nerve injury and can direct the selection of surgical methods and evaluate postoperative effects, and thus neural CEUS plays an important role in clinical diagnosis and treatment. When a nerve is injured and a scar forms, 2D ultrasound scanning sometimes results in incorrect judgement of nerve continuity. However, using CEUS to observe blood flow in the perineurium and epineurium can reduce the rate of misdiagnosis. During feasibility research on CEUS evaluation of peripheral nerve injuries and blood perfusion in neurogenic lesions, we found that blood perfusion of injured nerves plays a significant role in later repair and that the decrease in blood perfusion around the injured nerves may affect the regeneration and repair of nerves. CEUS can also identify neural lesions and cysts. Therefore, using CEUS imaging technology to evaluate early blood perfusion of injured nerves has significance and clinical value for neural repair and regeneration and later treatment.

5.3   Application of Visualized Interventional Ultrasound

Traditionally, nerve block often uses anatomic landmarks to pinpoint the target nerve in a blinded manner. Its effects are often impacted by anatomic variation, obesity, trauma, unclear surface landmarks due to individual anatomical differences, and poor compliance of patients, and as a result, it is unable to accurately pinpoint the target nerve.

Anaesthetic is not always injected into the ideal place for nerve block, which results in poor nerve block effects. Clinically, it is common to expand the anaesthesia scope by an increased drug dose to attain better block effects, but this is accompanied by commonly seen complications involving anaesthetic toxicity or accidentally injured vessels. Ultrasound visualization location technology with characteristics of non-invasion and visualization can clearly display the anatomical structure of the anaesthesia area and can guide the direction and depth of anaesthesia needling to perform accurate anaesthesia delivery and reduce the occurrence of anaesthesia complications. Therefore, this technology is clinically much more widely applied for nerve block. Ultrasound intervention technology has triggered a fundamental transformation of the treatment methods for peripheral nerve diseases and pain. It is easy to perform, less likely to cause, and has high accuracy, thus greatly reducing the rate of iatrogenic damage caused by peripheral nerve surgeries and blind paracentesis. This technology has brought revolutionary progress to ultrasonic diagnosis and location, guidance, treatment and biopsy for entrapment and injuries of peripheral nerve trunks and branches [3, 4].

With further research, ultrasound-guided nerve block has developed quickly. For example, 3D or 4D ultrasound neuroimaging is applied to guide nerve block, and real-time 3D imaging technology is applied to judge the drug's diffusion along nerves and vessels to guide and perform nerve block.

Currently, *ultrasound-guided nerve block* has been mainly applied to the following: (1) epidural block; (2) nerve block beside the thoracic vertebra; (3) nerve block of the brachial plexus; (4) nerve block of the lumbar plexus and femoral nerve; (5) regional anaesthesia for paediatrics; (6) nerve block at the neck and shoulders.

Ultrasonic visualization technology has been the most popular technology among patients for clinical treatment of minor injuries due to its convenience, practical application and easy acceptance. It is also an indispensable tool for physicians for diagnosis and treatment [5, 6]. The integration of visualization, diagnosis and treatment has been a trend for musculoskeletal ultrasound including ultrasound-guided treatment of subacromial bursitis, CEUS for rotator cuff injury, puncture and suction of bursa mucosa effusion and ganglion, block therapy for myotenositis, and peripheral nerve blocks (Figs. 5.5 and 5.6). Most patients prefer minimally invasive

treatment, and thus musculoskeletal intervention ultrasound has great potential.

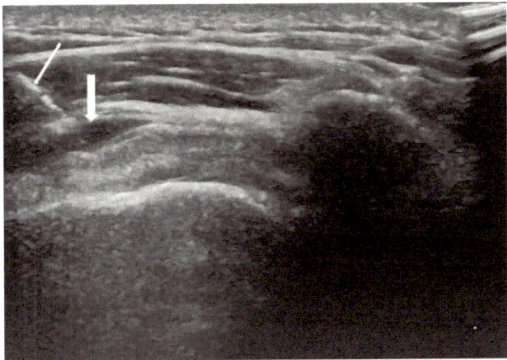

Fig. 5.5 Ultrasound-guided injection therapy for subacromial bursitis. Note: the thin arrow indicates the needle tip, and the thick arrow indicates the subacromial bursa

References

1. Bedewi MA, Nissman D, Aldossary NM, et al. Shear wave elastography of the brachial plexus roots at the interscalene groove. Neurol Res. 2018;40(9):805–10.
2. Cingoz M, Kandemirli SG, Alis DC, et al. Evaluation of median nerve by shear wave elastography and diffusion tensor imaging in carpal tunnel syndrome. Eur J Radiol. 2018;101:59–64.
3. Lee J, Kim K, Kim S. Treatment of a symptomatic cervical perineural cyst with ultrasound-guided cervical selective nerve root block: A case report. Medicine (Baltimore). 2018;97(37):e12412.
4. Dettori N. Choudu r H, Chhabra A. Ultrasound-Guided Treatment of Peripheral Nerve Pathology. Semin Musculoskelet Radiol. 2018;22(3):364–74.
5. Krishna Prasad BP, Joy B, Raghavendra VA, et al. Ultrasound-guided peripheral nerve interventions for common pain disorders. Indian J Radiol Imaging. 2018;28(1):85–92.
6. Guo XY, Xiong MX, Lu M, et al. Ultrasound-guided needle release of the transverse carpal ligament with and without corticosteroid injection for the treatment of carpal tunnel syndrome. J Orthop Surg Res. 2018;13(1):69.

Fig. 5.6 Ultrasound-guided cervical nerve block. Note: the white arrow indicates the middle scalene muscle, the yellow arrow indicates the anterior scalene muscle and the blue arrow indicates the needle tip

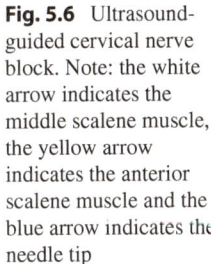
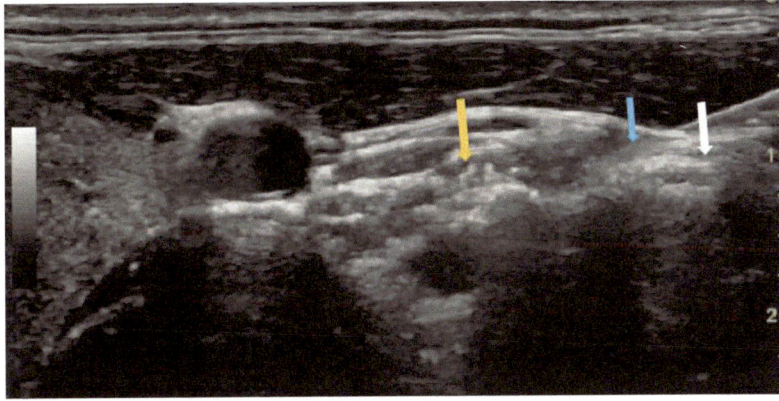

Correction to: Ultrasonography Diagnosis of Peripheral Nerves

Dingzhang Chen and Minjuan Zheng

Correction to:
D. Chen, M. Zheng (eds.), *Ultrasonography Diagnosis of Peripheral Nerves*,
https://doi.org/10.1007/978-981-15-2704-3

The original version of all the chapters were inadvertently published without video files. This has now been corrected and the video files are made available in the respective chapters along with its in-text citations.

The updated original version for this chapters can be found at https://doi.org/10.1007/978-981-15-2704-3